To:
Aggie & Dave

Stay Healthy!

Love

Jim

Your PROSTATE
Your LIBIDO
Your LIFE

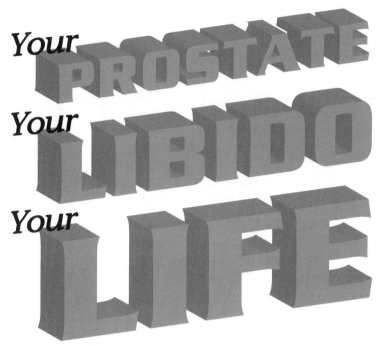

Your PROSTATE
Your LIBIDO
Your LIFE

*A Guide to Causes
and Natural Solutions
for Common Prostate Problems*

James Occhiogrosso, N. D.

Glenbridge Publishing Ltd.

Any information given in this book
is not intended to be taken as a
replacement for medical advice.
Any person with a condition requiring
medical attention should consult a
qualified practitioner or therapist.

Published by Glenbridge Publishing Ltd.
19923 E. Long Ave.
Centennial, Colorado 80016

Library of Congress Catalog Card Number: LC: 2007927035

International Standard Book Number: 978-0-944435-64-9

10 9 8 7 6 5 4 3 2 1

Table of Contents

Acknowledgments

It never fails to amaze me how much effort is involved in writing and producing a book. Aside from the author, many others offer input in the way of formatting, organization, and editing. These inputs are extremely valuable, and often precipitate rewriting entire sections to make them better. Many suggestions for making this book more valuable came from my good friend and racquetball partner, as well as noted author and scholar, Irvin D.S. Winsboro, Ph.D., Professor, Florida Gulf Coast University. His edits and suggestions made this book viable. I cannot thank him enough for his effort. I suppose now I will have to let him win at racquetball more often.

I would also like to thank Dr. Chip Shemansky, D.C., for his suggestions on the preliminary manuscript. Last, but certainly not least, I thank my wife Gerry, for her reading, corrections, and patience with her husband's addiction to writing books! A few books ago, I made her a promise that, one of these days, I would write our love story. Perhaps that will be my next project.

Preface

Discussion

There have been enormous technological advances in medical science in the past few decades. It is easier today to diagnose and treat many diseases than it has ever been. Some of the greatest modern benefits in healthcare, however, are not from these "technical goodies," but from the demands of informed consumers and the accompanying proliferation of organic foods and natural products.

Technical advances in diagnosing and treating complex diseases have also taken a quantum leap forward in recent years. However, statistics show that the incidence of many *serious*, chronic conditions—like diabetes, obesity, heart disease, and cancer—continues to increase. Thus, while we are steadily advancing our ability to treat these disorders, we are also losing the battle to prevent them!

Today, more and more people seek alternative methods to solve chronic health problems, as conventional medicine has limited resources in many of these areas. Informed healthcare consumers demand additional information beyond what their time-constrained and overworked doctors provide. And they demand more control over their treatment. In many cases, they refuse conventional treatment, sometimes wisely and sometimes disastrously.

Physicians sometimes mislead patients. Not because they mean to, but because they tend to treat symptoms instead of the underlying problems that cause them. Treating symptoms of a chronic condition can make the patient feel better. But without a coherent, long-term approach towards correcting the underlying cause, treating symptoms does little for a patient's overall prognosis.

And in certain cases, treating and suppressing symptoms may actually do more harm than good.

An analogy is quite simple. If you wear shoes that are too small, your feet will hurt. There are two possible solutions to this problem. You can treat the symptoms with painkillers to dull the pain, or you can attack the problem at its source by getting shoes that fit properly. It is obvious that the first solution—while it will likely work in the short term—does nothing to rectify the root problem. The focus of this book is to provide you with a working knowledge of the lifestyle and nutritional issues that cause prostate problems, along with some suggested approaches to help correct the underlying causes of these problems naturally.

In this book, I present many ways to change your lifestyle, your environment, and your diet to help you avoid or reverse prostate problems. This is basically a three-step process. The first step is to pay careful attention to your diet and environment with a goal of reducing exposure to environmental estrogens and other toxic chemicals. The second step is to change your lifestyle to include health-enhancing paradigms like regular exercise, and the third is to adjust your diet to include foods and supplements that enhance your overall health and specifically address any problems you are having with your prostate. All three steps have equal importance.

This book is based on scientific evidence gathered from medical studies published in peer-reviewed medical journals. I have deliberately avoided anecdotes from my own personal experience as well as the experiences of others. While I acknowledge that anecdotal evidence can never achieve the same level of certainty as randomized, double-blind, clinical studies, I also believe that multiple anecdotal reports as well as folklore often contain valuable information. It is difficult for researchers to obtain financing for clinical studies on natural products. This is due to the lack of profit incentive. Thus, folklore and anecdotal evidence, particularly the kind that has been around for hundreds of years, is sometimes the only information available. My contention is that multiple instances of anecdotal evidence, especially from different cultures, should be carefully examined and not dismissed simply because there is no conclusive clinical data.

While double-blind and reproducible scientific studies are certainly the standard to aim for, we must not forget that hard science often encompasses a single perspective, which is sometimes influenced by financial considerations. Frequently, results are not nearly as absolute as many in the medical profession would have us believe. This book is a good example of this. The etiology of prostate disease is controversial, and, as with any controversial subject, one can find numerous scientific studies that suggest different conclusions.

Why You Should Read This Book

If you have read this far, you likely have a prostate problem or you are concerned about developing one. There are many books available about prostate disorders. They discuss anatomy, medications, various prostate conditions, and conventional or alternative treatments. If you want that sort of information, this book is not for you. In this book, I assume that you know a little about the basics. I also assume that you want information that is more detailed about natural remedies and the science behind them that might help you. If you are lacking the basic information on this topic, I have provided a bibliography at the end of this book for additional reading.

The focus here is on the causes of prostate dysfunction. I provide information on nutrients, herbs, and lifestyle changes that can help alleviate common prostate problems. This book is not meant to provide detailed information on diagnosis or conventional medical treatments. Instead, it will give you a working knowledge of the factors that contribute to prostate dysfunction along with some well-researched, natural ways to overcome your problems. This information is for educational purposes only. It is not—in any way—intended to substitute for the advice or treatment of a medical professional. The reader should consult with a licensed medical practitioner in regard to any symptoms that require diagnosis or treatment. Many urinary, sexual, and other symptoms can indicate a serious problem, like prostate cancer.

If you were recently diagnosed with prostate cancer, take comfort that most prostate cancer is slow growing and has probably been with you for several years. A few hours spent learning more about your condition is unlikely to have a serious effect on your overall prognosis. I know of many cases of men diagnosed with prostate cancer who have rushed into aggressive treatment strictly on emotion. Such treatment is often impossible to undo and may cause serious side effects that you will subsequently regret. It is wiser to put your emotions aside and evaluate all your options before making treatment decisions.

What You Can Expect From This Book

This book is based on a natural approach to health. It provides information you can use to improve your overall health, and more specifically, offers a wealth of research related to improving prostate disorders naturally. Many elderly men suffering from prostate problems are unalterably wedded to medical practitioners who have little knowledge of nutritional healing and know even less about herbal medicine. It is important to remember that most pharmaceuticals came about as a result of scientists researching the action of herbs. Holistic health practitioners who use only natural substances can be a viable alternative for many chronic conditions. Such practitioners are professionals with extensive training in the effects of nutrients and herbs on body systems. This book presents natural ways to enhance prostate health, backed up by scientific research. Here you will find specific techniques for correcting lifestyle and nutritional deficiencies as well as a wealth of information on herbal remedies. Natural health techniques have worked for others with prostate problems. They can work for you, too.

If you are experiencing problems like erectile dysfunction, you may want to jump ahead to Chapter Nine and take the test called "The International Index of Erectile Function Test (IIEF or

IIEF-5)." Likewise, if you are having urinary difficulties, Chapter Eleven contains a test called the "International Prostate Symptom Score (IPSS)." You can take one or both of these tests now, and then retake them after you have made improvements in your diet and lifestyle. Perhaps you will be pleasantly surprised at the results. Printable versions of both tests are available on my website whose address is at the end of this section.

In this book I focus on the causes of prostate disease as well as the science behind recommendations you might see here and in other books and articles. Thus, this information is not only for you, but you may want to pass a copy along to your doctor. Some of the newer research referred to may conflict with what was taught in medical schools a few years ago. Your doctor may want to review the referenced studies.

Some information here may contradict other books. There are many items, particularly herbal combinations, that have enjoyed considerable popularity in the press, and on the Internet with little scientific evidence that they work. A man with a prostate problem, looking for information, can find himself subject to commercial advertising with amazing claims. Unfortunately, many of these claims have little backing in science or reality. The information in this book is the result of considerable research. If I could not find a reasonable amount of data to back an item, I have not included it.

I have provided a list of reputable websites that you can use to research herbs and other items in the appendix. Additional reference information, i.e., links to many other informational sites, the latest research on natural prostate healing, as well as links to purchase some of the herbs, supplements, and hormone creams mentioned in this book are also on my website.

What this book expects from you

The first few chapters of this book focus on defining the nutritional deficiencies and hormonal imbalances that appears to be at the root of most prostate dysfunction. If you read these introductory chapters carefully, you will gain an understanding of these items, many of which may apply to your own lifestyle. This will help you understand the reasons behind recommendations in the chapters that follow.

If you want to help yourself by using this book, you must commit to changing your life in several ways. Some of these changes are easy, while others may not be. You need not follow every suggestion. The more changes you adopt, however, the better you should feel and the more success you will have. If you incorporate the changes as a permanent part of your lifestyle, you will be well on the road to reversing your problem.

The information presented here has helped many men, including the author. I've written it to share some of my experiences and research with you in the hope of helping you get through a difficult time. I would love to hear your story too, so feel free to contact me through my website.

James Occhiogrosso, N.D.
http://www.ProstateHealthNaturally.com

Introduction

> We shall not cease from exploration.
> And the end of all our exploring
> will be to arrive where we started.
> And know the place for the first time.
> — *T.S. Eliot*

The words of T.S. Eliot above say it all for me. I suffered from various prostate problems for many years—trying remedies recommended by friends, Internet websites, and health food store clerks, while my problems continued to worsen. It was not until I began to explore the cause of my problems, and completed much of the research that resulted in this book, that I understood the real problem—and for the first time, knew the direction for my journey toward recovery.

How it All Began

The events that led to writing this book are somewhat convoluted. They began around 1990. I was fifty-two years old and preparing the final manuscript for my first book—a library of code routines for computer programmers. Back then my only interest, aside from my wonderful wife and family, was writing computer-programming libraries. I was also having some minor, but nagging, prostate symptoms. If anyone had told me then that sixteen years later I would be writing a book about prostate problems, I would have looked at them with total disbelief.

1

I sent my computer book to the publisher and then went to a doctor. My main complaints were in the area of a weak urinary stream, waking several times at night to urinate, erectile dysfunction (ED), and low libido. I was a bit embarrassed talking about it to my doctor, but I needed help. I had always been a very sexual guy, but suddenly, even when the desire was there, the mechanics were faltering. After several unproductive medical consultations, I began a search for something over the counter that might help. Back then, the current crop of ED drugs was only a fanciful dream. Most of the products I found were mechanical aids. If you have ever tried one of these, you already know what a serious damper they put on spontaneous lovemaking.

I continued writing computer books for a few more years, but my interest in that subject was waning. Meanwhile, prostate problems were demanding more and more of my attention. My urinary urgency had reached the point where I knew the location of every rest room wherever I went. A night of sleep—uninterrupted by the need to urinate—was but a memory. And, more often than not, lovemaking was mechanically impossible.

More doctor visits resulted in various tests, much embarrassment, and no results. One doctor told me I should learn to live with this kind of problem—after all, I was "getting older." Another told me the problem was probably psychological, and I should arrange a psychiatric consultation. A third, on learning I was an avid racquetball player, suggested I give up the sport. His reasoning was that at my age—if I wanted to have enough energy for sex—I would have to spend my energy more wisely. I think this particular doctor had his own problems with energy. He was only about forty years old, but a good seventy-five pounds overweight and breathing hard from a walk across the room. His attitude was that, at my age, I should grab my rocking chair, go sit on the porch, and wait to die!

That was the early 1990s. While rumors abounded about drugs that could fix ED, none were yet on the market. The FDA did not approve Viagra until March 27, 1998. Thus, my doctors had no magic pill to give me (although one did write a prescription for an antidepressant that I never filled). With their drug arsenal empty, they were helpless. I was in my early fifties, suffering from urinary urgency, nearly impotent, and damn unhappy about it! Fortunately (for my overall health), ED drugs were not available. If they were, I probably would have just gotten a prescription for one and gone on my way with that happy smile just like the actors in today's TV drug commercials. (We'll talk more about the damage that *"ignorance is bliss"* smile can do later.)

After a while I gave up on finding a medical solution, stopped trying various locker-room remedies, and began doing serious research. I bought stacks of books and researched libraries for information. Unfortunately, the Internet wasn't much of a resource back then. To my chagrin, I found lots of information about prostate problems (mostly cancer), but little about other problems like impotence. However, my research did lead to some books about nutrition that mentioned the subject in conjunction with nutritional deficiencies. This piqued my interest. Could it be that a nutritional deficiency was causing my problems? From nutrition books I went to general health books, then to herbology books, and then to more formal studies and a Doctor of Naturopathy diploma.

Of course, my larger goal was to correct my urinary urgency and erectile dysfunction, but I wound up getting an education about natural health. Meanwhile, the Internet came of age, making it easier to research medical information. I studied, improved my diet, ingested some specific vitamins, minerals, and herbs, and little by little I felt my prostate problems easing.

To make a long story short, I am writing this page just after my sixty-seventh birthday. I still play racquetball several times per week; I rarely wake more than once during the night to urinate; I don't have to stake out the location of every rest room before I take a trip; and my sex life is great. In short, my prostate (and overall health) is better now than it was nearly two decades ago.

An Emotional Issue

The title of this book evolved from my own emotions. When my prostate problems started, my sexual ability was one of the first things that suffered. Then, quality of life became an issue as every trip outside my home became a mental quest to remember the location of the nearest rest room. I found it amazing how fast a strong macho image is destroyed when one's sex life shuts down; it takes five minutes to start a urine stream; or you're in constant fear of wetting your pants. I realized then how much y*our prostate* affects *your libido* and *your life*, so the title seemed natural. My goal is to share my experiences in the sincere hope that they will be of significant help to my readers.

There are many books already on the shelf about natural solutions for prostate problems. Most devote much of their space to prostate cancer, are written primarily to educate men already diagnosed, and tend to concentrate on specific herbs or nutrients that can alleviate symptoms. While they provide pages of information on various treatments, little room is allotted for explanations regarding the origin of the disorder. Thus, their approach is similar to that of conventional medicine, except that herbal medications or "nutraceuticals" are recommended in lieu of "pharmaceuticals."

While this book does discuss prostate cancer, it focuses more on the issues often preceding that serious condition. Primarily, I examine the source of the problem, be it nutritional deficiencies, lifestyle, environment, or simply aging. The idea is that if you know the source, you can correct it, and in many cases eliminate or reduce the problem. Unfortunately for all of us, we have little control over aging. However, the suggestions here can help you reduce many of its effects, particularly regarding your sex life.

Much of the book is devoted to nutritional solutions for Erectile Dysfunction (ED or impotence) and Benign Prostatic Hyperplasia (BPH), also known as Benign Prostate Hypertrophy. Today, there are many pharmaceutical drugs available to alleviate both problems, but none addresses the underlying conditions that cause the problem.

In my opinion, long-term use of an erectile dysfunction drug is a prescription for disaster. While the drug will usually relieve symptoms of the problem, it leaves the underlying cause to fester and possibly grow into something more serious. As we will discuss in later chapters, ED is often the first indication of cardiovascular disease.

In addition, it is well-known that some drugs used to treat various chronic conditions—including BPH—can cause or exacerbate impotence. This poses a new dilemma, which is often solved with a prescription for another drug to counter symptoms caused by the first. I could continue this scenario, but I'm sure you already see where it's heading. If your doctor is quick to reach for the prescription pad, it is easy to fall into this trap.

Organization and Purpose

This book is organized into two parts. The first part, consisting of chapters one through five, reviews the causes and symptoms of various prostate conditions. Part II, which comprises the rest of the book, presents natural ways to alleviate prostate problems.

The first two chapters of Part I present an overview of the prostate and its potential problems. This overview is cursory and assumes you are already somewhat familiar with the basic anatomy. If you are not, you can find more detailed information in one of the books listed in the bibliography. Chapter Three discusses the multiple roles various sex steroid hormones have in relation to prostate problems. It explains, in simple terms, the main body processes that regulate hormone balance and how these processes become disrupted by aging and external factors. In Chapter Four I discuss how environmental problems and chronic diseases can cause or exacerbate prostate dysfunction. Chapter Five ends Part I with an in-depth discussion of the factors that lead to erectile dysfunction.

Part II, beginning with Chapter Six, looks at the many ways you can rebalance your body and start to reverse prostate dysfunction. This is where we examine how you can alter your lifestyle and nutrition to positively influence hormone balance and reduce negative effects on your prostate. I provide well-researched recommendations for common nutrients and herbal remedies. This analysis will help you to determine how to change your lifestyle and what substances may help your body reverse prostate problems. These natural solutions focus on giving your body the ammunition it needs to reverse your problems. Thus, you learn how to improve your overall health, and specifically the health of your prostate. My purpose is to show you how to provide your body with what it needs to heal itself, rather than just recommend substances to alleviate your symptoms.

It is better if you read this book in order, but if you want to get to the lifestyle and supplementation issues first, you can start with Part II and later come back to the beginning. However, by reading it in order you will have a better grasp of the reasons for many of the recommendations.

The bulk of this book is based on solid scientific evidence gathered from medical studies published in respected, peer-reviewed medical journals. A list of references is provided at the end of the book. There are areas in this book where my analysis or opinion may contradict that of some medical professionals. The origin of prostate problems is often controversial. Despite differences of opinion, this book is meant to help you and your doctor make informed decisions for your care. It is not meant to substitute for the advice of a competent medical professional.

If you are reading this book, it is likely that you—like many of us—want to avoid traditional medical treatments as much as possible, and that you want to take responsibility for your own health. So, that said, let's dig in and help you get healthier.

PART I

CAUSES AND SYMPTOMS OF PROSTATE PROBLEMS

Chapter One

Understanding The Problem

The prostate is subject to many problems. It is my belief that most of them can be traced to hormone imbalances in the body. I will use the terms "disease," "dysfunction," or "disorder" to refer to chronic conditions that affect the prostate or sexual function. Such problems can range from serious, like severe BPH or prostate cancer, to relatively benign, like low libido (lack of interest in sex) or erectile dysfunction.

Prostate cancer *can* be a serious, life-threatening condition, and as such, it is not the kind of problem you would normally self-treat. The key word here is *"can."* If you have been diagnosed with prostate cancer, keep in mind that it is often slow growing and *may* not require aggressive medical treatment. Here the key word is *"may."* Unfortunately, considerable differences of opinion regarding treatment exist within the medical profession. Based on the same information, one doctor may recommend an approach known as "watchful waiting," while another recommends immediate surgery or other aggressive treatment. The correct decision for you is one only you can make. And, making your decision may require consultation with several medical doctors as well as reviewing information on some of the many websites devoted to this illness.

This book is not intended to be a guide to curing prostate cancer. However, the nutritional and lifestyle issues it highlights are common to all types of prostate disease, including cancer, and are particularly relevant if you and your doctor have agreed to take a "watchful waiting" approach. (More on this later.)

If you are having a problem with your prostate, you are not alone! Prostate problems affect a significant portion of the male population. Considerable research in the past decade suggests that poor nutrition, lack of exercise, and environmental toxins are significant factors related to many chronic disorders, including those of the prostate.

Prostate disorders generally begin to present symptoms in men over forty, but they can appear at any time as a man ages. The cost to society of these problems is significant. Medical treatment can impose considerable burdens, resulting in impotence, incontinence, depression, relationship problems, lost workdays, hospitalizations, suicides, and other disruptions of normal lifestyle. Substantial benefits to society could be achieved if our focus was moved to a higher level of prevention of these disorders rather than simply treating them after they occur.

There appears to be many factors associated with the development of prostate dysfunction. Some of these are strongly linked to disease development and others are simply risk factors. Chief among the strongly linked agents is advancing age, with nutritional deficiencies and heredity following closely. While the incidence of virtually all prostate disorders increases significantly with aging, one's chances of developing serious prostate dysfunction increase directly with certain nutritional deficiencies. Of course, there is little you can do to forestall aging or overcome genetic factors, but there is certainly much one can do to minimize their effects. Nutritional deficiencies can be easily corrected once you confront them.

The Hormonal Factor

In examining studies of the various types of prostate disorders, there is a single underlying factor central to them all. Virtually all prostate dysfunction has a common issue—that hormones known as the "sex steroid hormones" are not in their normal balance. You have surely heard of the most famous of these—testosterone—but there are many others. In young men, most, but not all, of these hormones are higher than in older men. However, more is not always better. It is critically important that the levels of these hormones remain in relative balance.

Hormonal imbalance, in the form of an excess of some hormones and a deficiency of others is noted—in one way or another—in almost every study of prostate disorders. While many factors like nutrition, lifestyle, and genetics can be said to influence the development of prostate disease, their effects result in mediation of the body's collection of sex steroid hormones. Thus, a simple argument can be made that the cause of most prostate disorders is due to hormonal imbalance. While this statement is essentially true, it is also very broad and gives us little new information. An analogy would be to state that all cancer is due to a failure of the immune system. Again, the statement is true but conveys little usable information.

It is important to note that in much of the past literature and medical studies, roles of the various sex hormones were separated by gender. In some of the older literature, it was assumed that one gender produced certain hormones and the other did not. Recent studies have shown this to be untrue. Both sexes produce a full complement of all sex steroid hormones. Gender determines only their relative levels. For example, both men and women produce testosterone, but its level is considerably higher in a man than in a woman. The reverse is true of estrogen.

In the recent past, effects of so-called female hormones like the estrogens and progesterone (another so-called female hormone) have been shown to have male functionality.* Prior to the last decade, there was little research on these predominantly female hormones in men. Recently, imbalances in these hormones have been implicated in the development of various prostate conditions. While this book is about prostate disease in men, much of it can be extrapolated to breast disorders in women. The hormonal causes of various

_____

*For the purposes of this book, the term "estrogen" is used to refer to the group of predominantly female hormones consisting of estradiol, estrone, and estriol.

breast and prostate conditions are similar, and in many cases, both can be improved with the same lifestyle and nutritional approaches.

By examining how hormonal imbalances can lead to various prostate disorders we can better see how natural approaches to eliminate them can restore health. Such natural techniques include restoring hormone balance upset by aging, lifestyle, or other factors. This is accomplished by supplementing with natural hormones and/or herbal supplements, modifying nutritional profiles, eliminating external environmental pollutants, and changing lifestyle. Thus, understanding how the sex steroid hormones become out of balance is the first step towards reversing many chronic prostate problems.

A Note About Prostate Cancer

Most prostate conditions, including prostate cancer, are chronic problems. While prostate cancer can be life-threatening, it is certainly not in the same class as a massive heart attack or stroke. Advanced or aggressive prostate cancer is not the type of problem this book is about. While such problems can be helped with proper nutrition and herbal support, they always require the assistance of a medical professional and are not suitable for self-treatment.

Quite often, a diagnosis of prostate cancer is followed by recommendations for immediate treatment, either via surgery or radiation. In many cases, the diagnosis is paired with warnings of dire consequences if the recommended treatment is not implemented promptly. Keep in mind that prostate cancer is generally slow-growing. A short time spent evaluating different options is not likely to result in serious disease progression.

Many chronic illnesses, including prostate cancer, are the result of deterioration of a body system. All cancer results from a failure of your immune system. Your body is always producing cancer cells. A healthy immune system detects these wayward cells and destroys them before they can do serious damage.

Health often deteriorates slowly—in small, virtually unnoticeable increments. Sometimes, the deterioration is enough so that you are confronted with symptoms of serious illness. Other times, there are few symptoms, but you are told of a problem as a result of a laboratory test. Then you ask yourself, "how can I feel so healthy, yet be so sick?" The fact is, you didn't suddenly get sick, you suddenly started having symptoms, or got the bad news from your doctor!

Many so-called benign problems, when left untreated long enough, can turn into more serious ones like cancer. The Prostate Specific Antigen (PSA) test is a blood test typically used as an indicator for prostate cancer. It is not a highly conclusive test, as abnormal values can indicate problems other than cancer while normal values do not conclusively rule it out. There is much controversy regarding the PSA test. Some believe it is responsible for an increase in survival rates of prostate cancer, while others conclude that it simply skewing statistical survival rates because of the earlier detection of the cancer. In other words, is it improving the survival rate, or does the statistical improvement simply mean that men are living with knowledge of their cancer longer?

Typically, an elevated (abnormal) PSA leads to a prostate biopsy—a process where hollow needles are inserted into the gland and tissue is removed for analysis. This procedure can sometimes cause problems with large prostates, particularly if there is an infection present (prostatitis.)[1] If the prostate is enlarged and the biopsy is negative, the diagnosis is benign prostatic hyperplasia or BPH, which means abnormal prostate enlargement without any *detectable* cancer cells.

This is where conventional medicine fails us. A patient with a *benign* biopsy is sent home, happy with his *benign* diagnosis, and scheduled for another PSA and/or biopsy in six months or one year. Little is offered in the way of lifestyle modification or nutritional advice. Thus, the criteria that brought about the problem remain unaltered, and the patient is blissfully unaware that his condition may be progressing, and that the next biopsy—or the one after it—may not have such a pleasant outcome. Again, it is my strong belief that the time to address so-called *benign* problems is when they are first discovered—while they are still *benign*!

In my opinion, the term *benign* in BPH is a misnomer. In the medical studies I reviewed for this book, men with prostate cancer often had a history of BPH and/or prostatitis for several years before their cancer diagnosis. Thus, while there is no specific scientific proof that these conditions lead to prostate cancer, there is circumstantial evidence that they all originate from the same sources. The same can be said about erectile dysfunction. Again, in many of the studies I reviewed, men diagnosed with prostate cancer had a history of ED long before the diagnosis. The bottom line is that ED, BPH, and prostatitis—even though they are relatively benign conditions—are indicators that the prostate is not as healthy as it should be. Rather than wait for such conditions to develop into something potentially far worse, it is prudent to treat these conditions early.

Typically, conventional medicine approaches the more benign prostate problems with medication to alleviate symptoms. Again, while this solves the immediate problem, it does little to correct the cause. I believe the best approach is to rectify the problem at its source using natural techniques to improve the prostate's overall health. This may take longer, but the results are often permanent.

On the other hand, more serious conditions—like prostate cancer—often trigger treatments that could be classified as overkill. I have personally known several men who had small, nonaggressive prostate tumors, for which the treatment and its consequences were far more debilitating than the likely course of the disease!

Excessive apprehension can result in accepting treatment— alternative or conventional—of questionable value. In 1952 in *The Science and Practice of Iridology,* Dr. Bernard Jensen wrote:

> There is much being done in the healing arts today which coerces patients into doing what they should through fear.

More than fifty years later, Dr. Jensen's statement is still true, especially for a man when his sexual ability starts to wane, urination becomes difficult, his doctor tells him he needs a prostate biopsy, or he is told he has prostate cancer. His fear can easily lead him into accepting treatment that may not be in his best interest.

Fear is your enemy! It destroys your ability to make informed decisions and causes stress that exacerbates the problem.

Conventional Medical Approaches

Most of today's medical doctors are well equipped to handle life-threatening conditions. However, they are poorly trained to handle the less urgent, chronic problems that occur with increasing regularity in today's world. And they are virtually untrained in correcting the nutritional deficiencies that cause many of these chronic conditions. Unfortunately, many of today's medical doctors are also severely overworked. It is exceedingly hard for them to keep up with the latest advances in medical technology. Thus, finding one that is aware of the newest medical research as well as the latest information about herbology or nutrition is not feasible.

Pharmaceutical companies—for the purpose of developing and marketing drug products—finance a significant amount of today's medical research. Particularly in the United States, there is a dearth of good studies on the usefulness of herbal agents and other natural substances. Since these agents exist in natural form, they are not patentable, and thus of little interest to the profit-oriented pharmaceutical industry. Many people suffering from chronic conditions, including prostate dysfunction, who go to medical doctors only, have few options other than the drugs, surgery, or radiation treatments of conventional medicine.

The result of this is that proper nutritional supplementation, herbal support, and other health-enhancing or curative paradigms, are often ignored or marginalized in favor of conventional treatments. In the United States, organized medicine generally approaches prostate problems by attempting to alleviate symptoms with medication or correct them with surgery or radiation. Sometimes a condition has already caused extensive damage and such treatment is warranted. But many times, simply addressing the underlying cause of a condition can rectify it. Medication, radiation, and surgery do not address the chronic underlying causes of a problem, and thus they never completely eliminate it.

It is my contention that chronic prostate conditions do not appear suddenly like an attack of the flu, but rather they present themselves after years of poor lifestyle and nutrition. This argument is strengthened since most men are well over fifty when they first see a doctor about a prostate problem. If such conditions are caused by deficiencies of poor lifestyle and nutrition, then it is also my contention that a natural approach to correct such deficiencies can reverse some of the damage. Moreover, if the damage is not too severe, proper nutrition, lifestyle changes, and maybe a little herbal support, may even be able to reverse it all.

Many medical doctors who are unfamiliar with herbal and nutritional support for prostate problems tend to dismiss them as useless. If your doctor dismisses alternative techniques without even hearing about them, find another doctor! Some doctors have relationships with natural health professionals and will work with them to your benefit, but you may have to search carefully to find one. There are many ways to evaluate a doctor's potential to help you. Keep your eyes and ears open, read, and seek the advice of other health practitioners, particularly if you are being pressured to accept a particular treatment immediately. Not all medical doctors, and certainly not all urologists, are created equal. If your problem is not a serious one requiring immediate attention, herbal and nutritional support, along with some dietary and lifestyle changes, may be enough to reverse it.

Chapter Two

Prostate Anatomy and Types of Disease

Prostate Anatomy

The prostate is a walnut-sized gland positioned just below the urinary bladder and surrounds the urethra. (See Figure 1.) Its primary purpose is to provide seminal fluid for the male ejaculate during sexual intercourse. Secondly, it is the seat of a man's sexual ability. A properly functioning prostate gland and its surrounding nerve bundles are essential for sexual function. When the prostate mal-

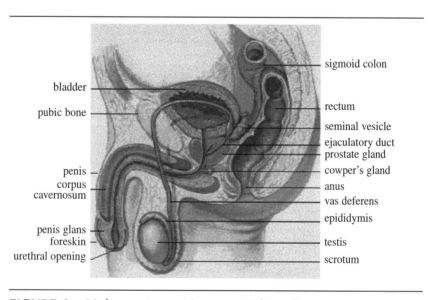

FIGURE 1. Male anatomy. Source: Wikipedia

functions, all sorts of symptoms arise, including erectile dysfunction, inability to reach an orgasm, pain on arousal or orgasm, and various urinary problems.

The urethra is a tube that passes through the prostate and provides a channel for urine to move from the urinary bladder through the penis and out of the body. Its secondary purpose is to carry prostatic secretions and seminal fluid containing sperm cells out of the body through the penis during sexual intercourse. Unfortunately, the strategic position of the prostate surrounding the urethra is why it causes men significant problems.

Usually, the prostate works seamlessly for much of a man's lifetime. But somewhere around the age of fifty, it becomes troublesome. Some of its problems, like benign prostate hyperplasia and erectile dysfunction, result mostly in discomfort and/or inconvenience. But others, like cancer, are quite serious and possibly life-threatening.

Unlike many other organs in the body that stop growing at an early age and rarely grow again, the prostate can initiate new growth later in life. It is this late-life growth that causes the bulk of prostate problems in middle-aged and older men. Enlargement of the prostate due to new growth can constrict the urethra, resulting in a reduced flow of urine. In severe cases, the excess growth can totally block the flow of urine through the urethra, resulting in a medical emergency. I refer to various prostate conditions generically as prostate disease, prostate disorder, or prostate dysfunction. Thus, these terms are interchangeable and include acute and chronic prostatitis (prostate infections), benign prostate hyperplasia (BPH), erectile dysfunction (ED or impotence), various prostate-related sexual problems, and prostate cancer.

Acute and Chronic Prostatitis

These are conditions where the prostate becomes infected and inflamed. Acute prostatitis is an infection that may be accompanied by severe pain, particularly in the area of the back and groin, inability to urinate, blood or pus in the urine, and a high fever. It is usually treated with antibiotics and/or other medications. Chronic prostatitis is a low-level infection of the prostate that may present few symptoms and may linger for years. There is no known cause for either condition, nor is it known whether they lead to more serious prostate disorders. There are some natural treatments that use herbal agents, but generally these conditions are hard to treat either conventionally or using alternative means. Neither condition is proven to be related to more serious problems and both may be helped by the techniques in this book that lead to a healthier prostate.

Erectile Dysfunction

This condition, frequently labeled "impotence," is a concern of virtually every man over the age of forty. It is defined as either an inability to reach sufficient penile hardness for vaginal penetration or inability to maintain an erection long enough to achieve satisfactory sexual intercourse. To achieve an erection and have satisfactory intercourse, the prostate must function properly. In the past, psychological factors were thought to be at the root of most male sexual problems. However, it is recognized today that only a small percentage of such problems are related to psychological conditions other than stress. A man's erection results from a complex combination of physical conditions, hormonal balance, nerve function, circulatory and overall health, as well as external stimuli to the brain. Anything that interferes with any of these pathways, including prescription or over-the-counter medications, can cause a problem, either temporarily, or permanently, in the case of a severe imbalance, chronic illness, or long-term drug use. The Association for Male Sexual Dysfunction recognizes over 200 drugs that may cause impotence.[1]

Orgasmic Dysfunction

Generally related to erectile dysfunction, orgasmic dysfunction (medically known as anorgasmia) occurs when a man is able to have a satisfactory erection, but unable to have a normal orgasm during sexual intercourse. There are several possible causes for this condition. Like most prostate disorders, it is strongly linked to advancing age. As men age, nerves in the penis tend to become less sensitive and chronic health conditions, particularly diabetes, can compound the problem by accelerating nerve deterioration. Orgasmic dysfunction can also be caused by psychological factors. Successful sex occurs in the mind as well as in the body. However, when psychological factors and nerve damage are ruled out, this condition is usually due to hormonal imbalances, particularly the testosterone deficiencies associated with aging. This is discussed in more detail in Chapter Eleven.

Benign Prostate Hyperplasia (BPH)

This is a nonmalignant enlargement of the prostate gland beyond its normal size. It is quite common in men over fifty. According to many experts, the incidence of BPH roughly parallels men's age groups. Approximately 50 percent of men suffer from it in their fifties, and this percentage increases to about 80 percent of men in their eighties.

For many men prostate growth begins in their late thirties with symptoms that are barely noticeable. Eventually though, the growth begins to interfere with prostatic or urinary function and symptoms appear. Symptoms of BPH typically include a frequent need or urgency to urinate, difficulty in starting or stopping urination, urine leakage, a weak, interrupted or split urine stream, blood in the urine, inability to void completely (urinary retention), and increased interruption of normal sleep due to the need to urinate (nocturia). Symptoms can also include erectile or orgasmic dysfunction. The most serious problem occurs when the condition progresses and interferes substantially with normal urinary flow. In severe cases, urinary retention can cause kidney problems, or the flow of urine can be totally blocked, requiring immediate medical intervention.

Prostate Cancer

This, of course, is the most serious of the prostate disorders. It represents a total failure of the body's immune system, and, while generally a slow-growing cancer, it can be life-threatening. Many urologists say that prostate cancer often presents no symptoms in its early stages. However, an aware man will notice various minor changes. Symptoms can include any or all of those of erectile dysfunction, orgasmic dysfunction, or BPH listed above. It is at this early time when natural intervention can achieve the greatest reversal of pending disease—before cancer is diagnosed. Unfortunately, many men, and their doctors, ignore these symptoms or write them off as normal aging until they become overwhelming. By then, it is often too late to reverse the problem.

While statistics for prostate cancer frequently produce headlines in the news media, lesser conditions, like BPH and erectile dysfunction, are typically underreported.

According to the National Cancer Society, more than 200,000 men are diagnosed with prostate cancer each year, and more than 30,000 die of it. However, the number of men quietly suffering with other problems may be several orders of magnitude larger. For example, a large study done a little more than a decade ago used a self-administered sexual activity questionnaire to determine the incidence of erectile dysfunction in 1300 male subjects between the ages of forty and seventy.[2] The report concluded that the combined incidence of erectile dysfunction ranging from minimal to total impotence was 52 percent of all men in this age range. Additionally, the prevalence of complete impotence tripled from 5 to 15 percent as subject ages neared seventy years. From this and other studies, it is estimated that the number of American men suffering from this condition is from twenty-five to well over thirty million, depending on the source. Thus, it certainly represents a significant problem.

Apparent Causes of Prostate Dysfunction

To date there is no "smoking gun" that has been proven to be the cause of prostate disease. In the study mentioned above (known as the MMAS study), subject age was the variable most strongly associated with impotence. It also concluded that a higher probability of impotence was directly correlated with heart disease, hypertension, vascular problems, diabetes, prescription medications, and indexes of anger and depression. Another finding of the MMAS study was that impotence was related to low blood levels of both the sex steroid hormone dehydroepiandrosterone (DHEA) and high-density lipoprotein (HDL) cholesterol (good cholesterol), and an index of dominant personality. Its final conclusion was that erectile dysfunction is a condition strongly associated with advancing age and has multiple determinants. Other studies have also confirmed a link between erectile dysfunction and high total serum cholesterol with low HDL/LDL ratios.[3, 4]

While the above discussion only relates to male impotence or erectile dysfunction, its conclusions can be extrapolated to include risk factors for other conditions of the prostate and several unrelated to the prostate.

I have taken the position that:

- Erectile dysfunction, benign prostate hyperplasia, and prostate cancer are all associated with the same risk factors;
- Erectile dysfunction may be the leading symptom of other, more serious disorders;
- Many of the risk factors for prostate disease are the same as those for other chronic conditions, such as diabetes, heart disease, vascular disease, and various cancers;
- These risk factors can be modified and reduced by changes in lifestyle and nutrition, intelligent natural hormonal balancing, and proper vitamin, mineral, and herbal supplementation.

The conventional medical approach to most prostate problems is similar to many other conditions—to alleviate the symptoms. In the case of prostate cancer that is confined to the gland and has not metastasized, an attempt is usually made to "cure" the disease by surgical removal of the prostate, implantation of radioactive palladium seeds within it, cryosurgery, or radiation.* However, in

---

*"Metastasized" means that the cancer has spread beyond the prostate gland. A discussion of metastasized prostate cancer is beyond the scope of this book.

many cases, the "cure" results in significant degradation of a man's quality of life and does not always affect the long-term prognosis.

Outside the United States, prostate cancer that is confined to the gland and deemed to be slow growing or unlikely to spread, is not always treated aggressively. In many cases, treatment consists of an approach called "watchful waiting," whereby the condition is monitored regularly without aggressive medical treatment. This is a reasonable approach, particularly with older men who are likely to die in ten years or less from other causes. However, while I strongly agree with initially withholding aggressive treatment in these cases, I do not agree with only monitoring and waiting, even with respect to older men. In my opinion, this passive approach simply allows time for the condition to reach a point where aggressive conventional medical treatment is mandatory! Far better is an approach targeted to improve overall health, particularly with respect to the prostate via proper nutrition and supplementation.

Most prostate disorders appear to develop along common pathways. Some studies have noted increased risk of prostate cancer, along with increased mortality in men diagnosed with prostate cancer, when the subjects had a prior history of BPH or prostatitis. Other studies did not find such an association. In this book, I have taken the position that the majority of prostate dysfunction is initiated by hormone imbalances caused by nutritional deficiencies, poor lifestyle, environmental factors, or generally poor health. I also take the position that ED, BPH, and prostatitis are not necessarily benign conditions, and that men suffering from them face a significantly higher risk of developing prostate cancer.* Some medical doctors may take exception to the foregoing, but this position is not contrary to the current stance of many experts.[5, 6, 7]

Prostate dysfunction is multifactorial. There are many nutritional and lifestyle issues that studies have linked to prostate disease, and, in particular, to prostate cancer. For many years the medical community has viewed high levels of circulating testosterone as

* This statement ignores erectile dysfunction problems induced by external factors such as: physical trauma, medications, chronic illnesses, or psychological disorders.

the "smoking gun" that causes prostate disease, particularly prostate cancer. Many experts believe that this simplistic approach is ignoring a growing tide of evidence that points to the contrary.[8, 9] In the chapters that follow, we will examine the multiple roles of the sex steroid hormones, particularly testosterone, and the effects that various nutritional deficiencies and lifestyle issues can have on hormone balance and disease development.

Chapter Three

The Role of the Sex Steroid Hormones

The human body is an amazingly complex mechanism. The more one studies it, the more one realizes how complex it is. Yet, all this complexity is for the most part controlled seamlessly with little conscious effort. Much of this control is due to the actions of minute amounts of substances called hormones. They circulate through the body producing powerful effects. While we understand many of the actions hormones produce, there are some whose actions are poorly understood. This chapter provides a simple discussion and overview of a group of hormones called the sex steroid hormones.

Hormone Basics

Hormones are the chemical messengers of the body. They are produced primarily in glands and organs that are part of our endocrine system.* However, other organs, such as the heart, can produce certain hormones as needed. Virtually every part of the body contains hormone receptors. Hormones and their receptors can be thought of as analogous to keys and locks. When the appropriate hormone (key) binds to a matching receptor (lock), it enables (unlocks) the

---

*The endocrine system consists of several glands that secrete hormones into the bloodstream. A discussion of this system is beyond the scope of this book. For more information, there are several books in the bibliography that provide detailed information.

receptor allowing the chemical message carried by the hormone to be transmitted to the internal mechanism of a cell.

Hormones circulate throughout the body in the bloodstream, searching for matching receptors to which to transmit their message. Receptors are found virtually everywhere in the body. Hormones are created as needed through interaction of various biochemical substrates like cholesterol and certain enzymes.* Once a particular hormone has transmitted its message, other enzymes break it down. There is a built-in feedback system that prevents the body from producing too much or too little of a given hormone. A healthy body maintains a constant homeostatic balance of virtually all its hormone levels.†

Each hormone has a detailed, specific message that it is designed to convey to an appropriate receptor. While many hormones and receptors are unique, some hormones perform similar functions and may be attracted to the same receptors. Conversely, some hormones can bind to multiple receptors. Most bind specifically, and most receptors attract only one type of hormone. When a hormone connects with an appropriate receptor on a cell, it unlocks the receptor, enters the cell, and transmits its chemical message. Within the cell, this triggers the action the hormone was designed to initiate.

Some hormones cause initiation of an action, and others can terminate it. A single hormone may find receptors in various areas of the body and convey a different message to each. For example, testosterone, which is one of the primary male sex hormones (or androgens), can bind with receptors in the brain to stimulate the desire for sex, receptors in muscle tissue to initiate growth, receptors on the skin to increase oil production, and receptors on prostate nerves during a penile erection.** Similarly, estrogen and progesterone,

---

* An enzyme is a protein that acts as an organic catalyst and is able to initiate or accelerate a specific biochemical reaction in the body.

† Homeostasis is the ability of the body to maintain itself in balance by constantly adjusting its internal processes.

** At puberty, young boys typically have problems with acne due to a rapid increase in testosterone triggering excess oil production in the skin.

typically deemed to be female hormones (and once thought to be produced only by females), can also bind to receptors on the prostate, initiating actions within the prostate to modulate its growth and function. Thus, the endocrine system, along with other organs that produce hormones, controls and regulates virtually every aspect of the body, from the rate at which the heart beats, to the desire and ability to have sexual intercourse.

Most prostate disease is hormonally sensitive, which means that hormone levels control or mediate it. For many years, conventional wisdom has been that the male hormone, testosterone, is the primary element that fuels prostate disorders like BPH and prostate cancer. We will examine this paradigm and challenge it in the light of recent research.

Hormone Hierarchy

The body produces many hormones. Some act directly on receptors, and some exist solely to control other hormones. Our chief focus are those that have direct involvement with the prostate, namely the sex steroid hormones.

Glands that contain many hormone receptors are said to be hormonally active. The prostate certainly fits this description. Virtually all of the sex steroid hormones have receptors on the prostate. These hormones are derived initially from cholesterol and then pregnenolone, from which the two major pathways of progesterone and dehydroepiandrosterone (DHEA) are created. The diagram below shows the major hormone pathways.

Both sexes produce all hormones shown, albeit males produce more testosterone (and other androgens) and less estrogens, and vice versa for females. Likewise, both sexes produce progesterone in differing proportions. The relative ratios between the male (androgens) and female (estrogens) help determine the external characteristics of men and women.

For simplicity, the intermediate steps in conversion of one hormone to another are not shown. Double arrows indicate that the

Major Sex Hormone Pathways

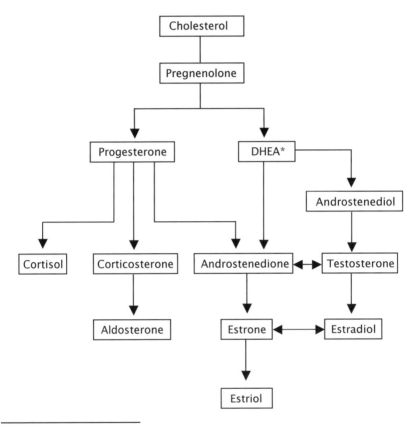

* DHEA = Dehydroepiandrosterone

conversion can go in either direction. As seen from the diagram, the critical male hormone, testosterone, can be produced through either of the two major pathways. The same is true of the critical female hormones, estrone, estradiol, and estriol. Estradiol (the most powerful estrogen) can be produced through the conversion of androstenedione and then estrone, or directly from testosterone. It is interesting to note that some hormones are produced from others and the conversion can go both ways. Others, like estriol, are "end points." They are not—to the best of our knowledge—converted.

Testosterone and Dihydrotestosterone (DHT)

Not shown in the diagram is an important intermediary hormone, dihydrotestosterone (DHT). It is a highly active form of testosterone that plays an important role in the development of various prostate disorders. DHT is an end point hormone that is derived exclusively from testosterone. As such, it cannot be converted to any of the more beneficial hormones.*

Traditionally, the medical establishment has viewed testosterone as the primary cause or accelerator of prostate cancer. The view has been that high levels of testosterone cause prostate cancer. This is based on research done in 1941 where castration was shown to slow or temporarily stop the growth and spread of prostate cancer. At that time, the relationship and role of DHT was not clear. Today, it is well-known that DHT is a potent mediator of abnormal prostate cell growth. However, much medical writing, particularly older studies and books, still support the theory that high testosterone levels are the cause of prostate problems. If this were so, young men, whose testosterone levels are high compared to older men, would be the primary group affected by prostate disease. In virtually all of the recent studies examined, high testosterone levels were not correlated to prostate disease.[1, 2] In fact, many studies found the opposite to be true. A recent study of disease-free, black, white, and Asian men found that levels of total and free testosterone were lowest in the black men, intermediate in the white men, and highest in the Asians.[3] This is in stark contradiction to the known risk levels of high, medium, and low (respectively) for prostate cancer in these groups. Coincidentally, the ratio of DHT to testosterone in these groups was highest in black men, intermediate in white men, and lowest in the Asians, which is more in line with each groups known risk level.

---

* You may have heard that excess DHT causes hair loss (balding) in men. You may have also heard that excess DHT may cause BPH or fuel prostate cancer cell growth. These statements all appear to be supported by the research.

Development of Prostate Problems

Excess DHT appears to stimulate abnormal tissue proliferation in the prostate. Testosterone is converted to DHT by the action of an enzyme called 5-alpha-reductase. A high level of this enzyme results in a higher level of conversion, and consequently, in increased growth of prostate tissue. Conversely, low levels of 5-alpha-reductase are associated with small or normal prostates.[4]

Increased levels of 5-alpha-reductase may cause an imbalance in two genes that regulate normal cell growth—the p53 and bcl-2 genes. The p53 gene inhibits cell growth and the bcl-2 gene activates it. Cancer can occur when the balance between these genes is upset and the bcl-2 gene dominates. The action that causes this is not known, but there is a suggestion that it may be related to increasing levels of 5-alpha-reductase, or deficiencies in certain micronutrients. A recent article in the *Journal of the American Medical Association* discussing these genes indicated that estradiol turns on the bcl-2 gene and progesterone inhibits it.[5] In addition to the negative effects where excess 5-alpha-reductase increases conversion of testosterone to DHT, recent studies indicate that estradiol—either alone or synergistically with various other androgens—assists in the development of prostate disease.[6] Like DHT, estrogen production is mediated by the action of an enzyme. In this case, the enzyme is called "aromatase." High levels of aromatase result in increased conversion of testosterone to estrogen and thus an imbalance in the testosterone to estrogen ratio.

Recent studies have indicated that while DHT is widely acknowledged to be a primary agent in the development of prostate disease, the estrogens, particularly estradiol, are also significant.[7, 8] Some functions previously ascribed to various androgens are now attributed to the action of estrogen in the prostate. High levels of the 5-alpha-reductase and aromatase enzymes result in elevated levels of DHT and estradiol and lowered testosterone levels. The latest research appears to indicate that the increase in conversion of testosterone to DHT and estradiol, rather than the overall testosterone level, is a primary factor initiating many prostate problems.

This contradicts some widely held beliefs in the medical community. For many years, the prevailing wisdom has been that excess testosterone was the most important mediator of prostate disease. A growing body of current research contradicts this, but long entrenched beliefs are often hard to overcome.

Both DHT and estradiol are necessary for proper functioning of the prostate, but their levels can become skewed due to nutritional deficiencies or lifestyle/environmental issues. When they become unbalanced with respect to the other sex hormones, the problems start. It is quite easy to conclude that the primary cause of most prostate conditions is a long-term, underlying metabolic imbalance. This imbalance causes increased conversion of normally beneficial testosterone to its more active form, DHT. Simultaneously, it increases sensitivity of the prostate to the estrogens. Both this increased conversion of testosterone to DHT, and an increased sensitivity to the estrogens, particularly estradiol, appear to be significant agents in the development of prostate disease. Thus, to prevent or ameliorate most prostate problems, including cancer, we need to examine the environmental, nutritional, and lifestyle factors that contribute to this metabolic imbalance—and most importantly, find ways to correct it.

Testosterone and Sex Hormone Binding Globulin (SHBG)

As mentioned earlier, the highest risk factor for prostate dysfunction is advancing age. It is well-known that males experience a decline in androgens, primarily testosterone, as they age. As a man ages from fifty to seventy, his testosterone level can decline as much as 30 to 50 percent.[9, 10] If he started out on the low side in his earlier years, this decline can be more pronounced. As this drop in testosterone occurs, a simultaneous age-related increase occurs in a protein called "sex hormone binding globulin" (SHBG).

Virtually all hormones exist in the body in two forms, free and bound. Only free hormones are active. Bound hormones are paired with SHBG and cannot bind with receptors. The net effect is that the age-related decrease in total testosterone is magnified by this increased binding to SHBG, resulting in a lessened amount of free testosterone.

When testosterone becomes bound to SHBG, its ability to attach to receptors is inhibited. Since only free testosterone can deliver its hormonal message to prostatic receptors, a rise in SHBG is significant. It results in symptoms of low testosterone, even though total testosterone levels may appear normal. (See box below for some notes about what is normal.) In addition, lowered levels of free testosterone and increased levels of SHBG tend to magnify the effects of estradiol. Aging also causes a slight rise in estradiol, which compounds the problem. Some research suggests that increased levels of estradiol activate the liver to make more estradiol.[11, 12, 13] Thus, the ratio of most of the androgens to estrogens is altered significantly, setting the scene for prostate dysfunction. These combined effects of elevated estradiol and SHBG, along with corresponding lowered levels of free testosterone have a profound effect and are significant contributors to the development of BPH and other prostate conditions as a man ages.

What is Normal?

Normal testosterone levels are derived from a sampling of a large number of presumed healthy men of various ages. The results are separated into age groups and averaged for each group. Normal levels of testosterone vary by about 5:1 from high to low. Older men are generally at the lower end of the range. Based on this, it is considered normal for older men to have lower levels of testosterone. However, in many of the studies reviewed for this book, it appears that prostate problems occur more frequently in men with relatively low testosterone levels. Perhaps we need to redefine our perception of *normal*. It is evident that *normal* may be quite different from *optimal*.

Conventional Approaches

Treatments to alleviate symptoms of BPH and to slow prostate growth generally seek to reduce circulating testosterone or DHT levels. For example, the drug Finasteride, (Propecia, Proscar), that is used to treat BPH, works by blocking the 5-alpha-reductase enzyme, thus blocking conversion of testosterone to DHT. In some cases, it can help shrink the excess tissue of BPH. However, in many cases it simply does not have the desired effect, which indicates that there are other mediating factors. It also has unacceptable side effects. One of its most common side effects is loss of sexual libido or ability, and consequential erectile dysfunction. Since most men value their sexual ability, the drug is often counterproductive. In many studies, herbal supplementation was found to be superior to Finasteride for symptomatic relief of BPH. (See the sections on phytoestrogens and beta-sitosterols in Chapter Eight.) Another treatment is to inhibit the action of the aromatase enzyme that converts testosterone to estradiol. This lowers overall estradiol levels and thereby increases the testosterone to estradiol ratio.

Progesterone and DHEA

As shown in the diagram, both progesterone and DHEA are testosterone precursors. The previous accepted belief that the prostate was responsive only to androgens is now known to be incorrect. The prostate is rich in receptors for progesterone, in addition to its androgen and estrogen receptors.[14, 15] While both estrogen and progesterone were previously thought to be specifically female, with little effect on the prostate, quite the opposite is true. This new paradigm is significant.

Progesterone, in addition to its own properties, has profound effects on the availability of all the other sex hormones. A deficiency in progesterone inherently results in deficiency of some of the others. As a man ages, his progesterone production decreases, resulting in a corresponding decrease in his levels of testosterone.

At the same time more of his available testosterone is converted to DHT and estradiol.[16, 17] The end result is that the relative ratios of estrogen to progesterone, and estrogen to testosterone increase. This allows more estrogen (particularly estradiol) to reach receptors on the prostate, thereby increasing its overall effect. Some studies have also found that estradiol reduces the body's clearance of DHT from the prostate, thereby compounding the problem. Similarly, on the other major pathway, the level of DHEA also drops, resulting in an additional decrease in testosterone levels, again compounding the problem. Many recent studies have found that both low levels of DHEA and testosterone correspond directly to prostate problems. Thus, the age-related drop in progesterone, DHEA, and testosterone, and the relative rise in estrogen and SHBG levels, results in increased risk for prostate problems. Coincidentally, excess estradiol is also known to be a key player in abnormal breast tissue proliferation. This is one reason older men frequently have enlarged breasts.

The significance of the drop in progesterone and increase in the ratio of estrogen to progesterone cannot be ignored. Studies indicate that progesterone increases the effects of the p53 gene that inhibits cancer growth and decreases the effects of the bcl-2 gene that accelerates it.[18, 19] The same studies (and others) also found that estradiol has the opposite effect on these genes. Thus, the observed drop in progesterone, combined with the increased effect of estrogen, can be a prescription for disaster.

Note that the above discussion refers only to natural or bio-identical progesterone. Compounds called progesterone produced by the pharmaceutical industry, and generally known as "progestins," are similar in structure to natural progesterone, but differ profoundly in their effects on the body. Most researchers are well aware of the significantly different effects of natural progesterone and synthetic progestins. However, the pharmaceutical industry often links the terms "progestins" and "progesterone." Printed literature typically makes no distinction between the two. As a result, many medical practitioners—and the general public—believe they are the same. They are not! They are structurally different and have profoundly different effects on the human body.[16, 17, 20]

Progesterone, as referred to in this book, represents only the hormone that is identical to that produced by the body. On a similar note, the age-related drop in estrogens referred to above relates only to natural estrogens produced by the body, not synthetic estrogens or xenoestrogens (also called pseudoestrogens) introduced into the body via prescription medication or through the environment. These are discussed in the next chapter.

Effects and Symptoms of Hormone Imbalance

Many changes take place in a man's body as he ages due to changes in the levels of circulating hormones. TV commercials may lead you to believe the only effect is a decline in testosterone. Of course, in these advertisements, this deficiency can be corrected with a quick visit to your doctor and a testosterone shot or patch. However, the picture is not that simple. While it is true that testosterone levels decrease with age, there are other substances and hormones that decrease or increase at the same time. It is the balance between them that is critical, not the absolute numbers.

Although both men and women experience lowered levels of certain hormones as they age, symptoms of the decline differ significantly. With women, the drop is marked by the physical end of their menstrual cycle and is called menopause. It is mostly due to a decrease in estrogen levels, along with almost total cessation of the production of progesterone, and is marked by symptoms like hot flashes, night sweats, and general irritability. Men have a similar drop in sex steroid hormones, but do not have an obvious physical marker for the condition, as do women, and their symptoms are more subtle. The condition, however, is quite real, and many professionals now use the terms "andropause" or "PADAM" an acronym for "Partial Androgen Deficiency of the Aging Male" to describe it. In the past, it was thought that andropause was caused primarily by a drop in the level of the man's most potent sex hormone, testosterone. However, there are also accompanying drops in other hormones, namely DHEA and progesterone, as well as increases in

SHBG and estradiol. The age-related changes in relative ratios of these hormones have a direct effect on the prostate, the libido, and a host of physical characteristics.

The decrease in the androgen to estrogen ratio is the primary source of the symptoms many aging males experience. Its symptoms include: reduction of sex drive, erectile dysfunction, uncomfortable or painful ejaculation, reduced ejaculate, difficulty achieving orgasm, blood in the urine or semen, loss of muscle mass, lowered energy levels, decreased exercise tolerance, depression, increased urinary urgency or frequency, and breast enlargement. While some of these symptoms can be the result of minor problems, they may also accompany serious problems and should be evaluated. By maintaining overall health and hormone balance, many men can alleviate these symptoms and restore youthful vigor.

Summary

As men age, their levels of estradiol and sex hormone binding globulin (SHBG) gradually rise, while the levels of progesterone, DHEA, and testosterone usually decline significantly. At the same time, the enzyme 5-alpha-reductase that converts testosterone to DHT also rises, as does the aromatase enzyme that converts testosterone to estrogen. The net effect is an increase in the estrogens and DHT, and a decrease in androgens, with a marked lowering of free testosterone. As the ratio of estrogens to androgens increases, so does the incidence of prostate disorders. A large number of studies have linked imbalances in estrogen to androgen ratios to the development of both breast and prostate cancer.

Aside from normal aging, which is beyond our control, there are many lifestyle and nutritional issues that can cause additional estrogen production or initiate a reduction in androgens. For example, excess fat tissue produces estrogens. An overweight or obese man can have significantly higher estrogen levels than a man of normal weight. Alcohol consumption, smoking, and many other environmental factors can exacerbate age-related hormone imbalances.

In contrast to aging, external factors are certainly controllable, at least to a degree, if one is willing to make the effort to do so. In Part II of this book, we examine ways to correct the influence of some of these environmental factors.

Chapter Four

Other Factors Affecting Hormone Balance

Each factor that initiates an imbalance in the body's sex steroid hormones contributes to the development and progression of prostate disease. When a man's hormone levels become skewed from the norm, dysfunction is not far behind. Hormone balance is influenced by many factors. Among them are advancing age, genetic predisposition, nutrition, medications, poor health, and the environment.

While aging and genetic predisposition are beyond one's control, external factors are not. Poor nutrition can cause an increase in estrogen production and a corresponding decrease in testosterone. Lifestyle issues like smoking and excessive alcohol consumption can also skew hormones unfavorably. Chemical agents that exert estrogen-like effects on the body can cause severe imbalances in hormone levels. Fortunately, these environmental and lifestyle issues can be modified, and thus their influence lessened.

As mentioned previously, estrogen levels normally tend to increase as men age. However, if advancing age were the only event mediating this increase, the effects would have considerably less impact. Unfortunately, many products in our environment and food supply, when absorbed by the body, mimic the effects of estrogens produced by the body. These artificially induced increases in estrogen levels can exceed those of normal aging, adding considerably to the imbalance in the body's estrogen to androgen ratio. In simple terms, this can be called an "estrogen overload" condition. It is a major player in the development of many disorders including several types of cancer.

Thus, aside from normal aging, lifestyle and nutritional issues can cause additional estrogen overload or a reduction in androgens. Since age-related rises in estrogen occur at the same time as androgen levels decrease, estrogen introduced into the body by the environment adds to imbalances caused by aging, increasing the risk of developing prostate dysfunction.

Environmental Estrogens
(Xenoestrogens and Phytoestrogens)

Many modern chemicals have estrogen-like effects when introduced into the body. These various compounds are derived mostly from petrochemical products. They bind with estrogen receptors—particularly those in the prostate—and mimic the action of the body's natural estrogens. These environmental agents are generally known as *xenoestrogens* or *pseudoestrogens*—terms coined by various researchers to describe chemicals appearing in our environment and food chain, which produce estrogen-like effects on the body.* Many of these chemicals are known in the scientific community as "endocrine disrupters," indicating their ability to disturb the human hormonal system.[1]

Plant sources also produce chemicals that can mimic the effects of estrogen. These are called phytoestrogens. They are found in many plants and herbs. Estrogen-like compounds from plants are generally self-balancing. While they mimic many actions of estrogen, they do it weakly, and do not usually cause ill effects. More importantly, they tend to negate some of the harmful effects of other estrogens without raising estrogen production in the body. A common herb for treating the hot flashes of menopausal women is black cohosh. It is an herb rich in phytoestrogens that helps a woman's body via two actions. The first is by supplying estrogen-like compounds that help

---

* The prefix "xeno" comes from the Greek word "xenos," which translates to odd, different, or strange.

reduce the effects of the menopausal drop in estrogen, and the second by supplying progesterone-like sterols that sensitize estrogen receptors in the body resulting in a lessened need for estrogen.[2] The same relative action occurs in a man's body when phytoestrogens bind with receptors on and around the prostate gland.

The story is quite different for xenoestrogens. They are chemical agents that mimic the deleterious effect of estrogens. Their inorganic composition disables the body's control mechanism. Virtually all plastic items contain these estrogen-like compounds, and our modern environment is overwhelmed with plastic. If you think this means the plastic wrap covering virtually everything bought in today's modern supermarkets is adding xenoestrogens to your body—you are right on target! This and other similar sources leach these estrogen-like compounds into the food we eat in ways that were unheard of years ago. Unlike phytoestrogens, xenoestrogens are not self-balancing. They strongly mimic negative effects of estrogen in the body. In the past few decades we have seen an increased incidence of various hormonally sensitive cancers like breast and prostate cancer. It is quite feasible that part of this increase is due to today's ubiquitous plastics products and their analogs.

For example, the pesticide DDT was banned about thirty years ago in both the United States and Europe. In a recent study, toxicologist Corinne Charlier of Sart Tilman Hospital in Liège, Belgium, found that women with breast cancer were five times more likely to have DDT residues in their blood.[3, 4] Like many other petrochemical compounds, DDT mimics the action of estrogen and related hormones. Until recently, a petrochemical called DES was used as an agent to fatten beef cattle prior to slaughter. DES is also known to have estrogenic effects on the body. While it is no longer used extensively, the practice of feeding beef cattle estrogenic-like compounds to fatten them for slaughter continues today. The same practice is also used with poultry and other commercially produced food animals. Presumably, petrochemicals used today for this purpose are less dangerous than DES, but there is no evidence that they are without danger.

In addition to the estrogens from animal products, xenoestrogens leach into the food supply from the very containers that the food is packaged in, as well as from the use of pesticides, detergents, personal care products, and other common items of petrochemical origin. Another source is the unenlightened preparation of food, by using plastic containers and utensils while cooking or heating foods in microwave ovens.*

The entry of these environmental estrogen-like components into the body causes significant problems. When one of them is introduced, all the body can do is decrease its internal estrogen production. Many built-in feedback loops normally help the body keep its hormones in proper relative balance. However, when the incoming hormone load is excessive, all the body can do is stop internal production of the offending hormone. If the level still exceeds that needed for balance, the owner of that body is in big trouble indeed! Evidence in a multitude of recent studies suggests that the presence of excess estrogens, particularly xenoestrogens, is a strong risk factor for developing prostate cancer. Experts have hypothesized a similar analogy for breast cancer.

Reducing Estrogen Overload

Estrogen in the body comes from two sources. One is the body's production of estrogen and the other is external from food or the environment. To avoid overwhelming the body with estrogenic-like compounds is, to say the least, a formidable task. Excess estrogen is a major player in the development of hormonally sensitive cancers, like prostate and breast cancer. To reduce your risk, you must take steps to lower production of internal estrogens and minimize exposure to external xenoestrogens. Estrogen is produced internally by

---

* Microwave ovens use high-energy radiation to cause molecular heating in food. This energy generally passes through the container holding the food. This combination of high energy and heat can force xenoestrogens from the container into the food. If you use a microwave oven, it is prudent to avoid using plastics or plastic wraps in it.

the endocrine system and by adipose (fat) tissue. Thus, simply reducing the amount of fat tissue in the body helps to reduce circulating estrogen levels. This is especially true if a person is overweight or obese.

Pesticides and herbicides are prime sources of environmental estrogens. By purchasing only organically grown fruits and vegetables, you can reduce this exposure path considerably. Such products not only taste better, but studies have shown they contain more nutrients. Also, while they are not completely free of pesticides and herbicides, the concentration of these toxins in them is significantly lower.

Phytoestrogens, the weak estrogen-like compounds found in plants, can also be used. They bind with estrogen receptors in the body, blocking some of the effects of the other estrogens. This natural technique reduces the negative effects of both external xeno-estrogens and estrogens produced by the body. It also helps to normalize your estrogen to testosterone ratio. This is discussed in more detail in Chapter Nine.

The High-Fat, Red Meat Diet

Several studies have found a strong correlation between a high-fat diet and prostate disease, particularly prostate cancer. Conversely, others failed to link fat in the diet with prostate problems. Generally, in studies that linked prostate cancer to high-fat consumption, the fat came from animal sources like red meats. In those that failed to link fat consumption with prostate cancer, fat sources were mainly plant based. This is significant! Most animal fat consumed in westernized countries comes from animals fed grains and hormones to stimulate fast growth. Consuming meat from such hormone-laden sources increases circulating estrogen levels in both men and women. And, as we have seen, high estrogen levels correlate positively to breast and prostate disorders—especially cancer. Studies have also associated a high animal fat diet with other cancers.

The obvious fact is—not all fats are created equal. A 1975 study over thirty-two countries concluded that prostate cancer mortality was highly associated with total fat consumption.[5] In 1986, another study confirmed these results, and further determined that the link to high-fat diets was from the intake of animal fat rather than vegetable fat.[6] This association to a high animal-fat diet was quite evident, not only for prostate cancer, but for other cancers, including breast, ovarian, and colon cancer. According to the 1986 study, the correlation with breast cancer was particularly strong in postmenopausal women. International comparisons strongly suggest a reduced risk of these cancers in areas where the major source of dietary fats are from plant, rather than animal sources. A recent study of diet and prostate cancer in China—an area noted for its lower incidence of prostate disease than the United States—also confirmed the relationship between a diet high in animal fat and prostate disease.[7] Thus, both breast and prostate cancer have a positive correlation with high consumption of animal fat in the form of meat and milk products.[8]

In many countries, animals for human consumption are fed diets of grain and other items treated with hormones to enhance growth and thus the market price of the meat. All mammals, including humans, tend to store hormones like estrogen in fat tissue. When you eat the meat of animals fed with hormone-laden grain you get a dose of estrogen along with your hamburger! Animal fat also seems to have a unique ability to cause the body to produce more estrogen.

As a specific example, the diet of many people living in the Mediterranean area has a common ingredient of thin oils like olive, fish, and peanut. All of these items have high fat content. While this population has a high-fat diet, the bulk of the fat intake is from plant rather than animal sources. This area is noted for a particularly low incidence of prostate and breast problems, particularly cancers.

On the other hand, a contradiction occurs when one looks at studies of the Inuit peoples that inhabit Arctic regions. While they consume more animal fat in their diets than most other cultures on the planet, they are generally free of the prostate disorders that plague westernized countries. Significantly, the animal fat they consume comes almost entirely from wild, rather than farm-raised, animals. Wild animals are not subject to a diet of hormone-laden grains, and this is reflected in their meat.

Nearly all of the studies suggest that fat consumption from plant, rather than animal sources, appears to be protective. Western experts have been advocating low fat consumptions for years, but the recommendations usually do not distinguish between types of fats. Animals fed a diet alien to them cannot maintain a level of good health. The result of feeding grass-fed beef cattle hormone-laced grains, is unhealthy animals. And eating the meat of these animals is detrimental to the health of those who consume it. Cattle raised for milk production have essentially the same problem. Cows are fed hormones to maximize milk output. Dairy products made from hormone-laden milk also appear to increase the risk of prostate disease.[9, 10] Several studies have linked high-fat, high-calcium (in excess of 1500 mg/day) diets, primarily from dairy products, to prostate cancer progression. While calcium is necessary in the human diet, there are far better sources for it than dairy products.

Another problem with farm-raised animals is that they are subject to crowded living conditions. This invariably increases their susceptibility to disease, and they need to be fed antibiotics to keep contagious illnesses under control. So, when you eat the meat of farm-raised animals, you may also get some unneeded antibiotics. This comes in addition to the dose of unwanted hormones discussed earlier.

The meat of farm-raised animals has other problems, such as an imbalance in omega-3 and omega-6 fatty acids and excessive estrogen-laden fat tissue. Beef cattle are grass-eating creatures. Organic beef typically comes from grass-fed rather than grain-fattened cattle. Cattle fed a diet of grains laced with hormones yield meat that has a skewed ratio of the essential fatty acids (EFA's), omega-6 and omega-3. Typical is 20:1 omega-6 to omega-3. The human body is programmed for an omega-6 to omega-3 ratio of approximately 1:1. Organically raised, grass-fed beef typically has a ratio closer to the body's target, which is better for human consumption. Such meat also contains less overall fat and is less of a storage medium for estrogens. Organic beef as well as meat from other organically raised animals is usually certified to be hormone free, indicating that no hormones were used to artificially stimulate the growth of the animal or increase its fat content.

Suffice to say that, if you are trying to correct or avoid prostate problems, you would be wise to limit your intake of meat and meat products from farm-raised animals. It is also wise to eliminate most dairy products, particularly cheeses and milk. Most health food stores carry a line of organically raised beef, chicken, and other meats including bison. The suppliers guarantee these products are produced without the use of antibiotics or hormones. Remember, cattle are grass-eating creatures. Look for *grass-fed, free-roaming,* and *hormone-free* on the label.

Dietary Problems and Obesity

There are many factors other than consumption of fat from hormone-fed animals that may effect or cause prostate problems. Typically, people who consume the most fat and red meat also eat large amounts of highly processed foods and sugars and the least amount of fruits and vegetables, thus depriving themselves of many valuable nutrients and enzymes. These people typically suffer from the hormone-skewing effects of their high-fat diet, along with vitamin and/or mineral deficiencies and digestive problems.

In several studies, a high animal fat, low fruit and low vegetable diet was conclusively associated with an increased risk for prostate cancer, while a diet rich in fruits, vegetables, and other plant products had a protective effect against this cancer.[11, 12, 13, 14] Several studies also show that men with diets high in fiber have a lower incidence of prostate cancer, and one found that men with prostate cancer who ate green and yellow vegetables each day, had lower mortality rates from their cancers.[15, 16, 17]

Overweight and obese men are subject to an increased incidence of many health problems, including those of the prostate. In recent studies, obese men had significantly increased risk of developing aggressive prostate cancer.[18, 19] Adipose (fat) tissue stores estrogen and recent studies also confirm that it produces estrogen. Thus, excess fat in the diet results in more fat tissue, which in turn causes increased estrogen storage and production. The net result is an increase in the estrogen to androgen ratio. This action alone is associated with prostate dysfunction. In addition, obese individuals also tend to have other health issues like diabetes, high blood pressure, high cholesterol and triglyceride levels, and impaired immunity, all of which can exacerbate prostate problems.

Nutritional Deficiencies and the Standard American Diet (SAD)

It is hard for many people to believe that there could be anyone suffering from nutritional deficiencies in our society. Unfortunately, deficiencies are quite common. According to a considerable amount of research done in the past two decades, middle-class people living in westernized countries—particularly the United States—suffer from considerable nutrient deficits. Chief among these are mineral deficiencies, with vitamin and enzyme deficiencies not far behind.

The cause of this is multifactorial, but two factors predominate. First, the diet of many Americans consists of highly processed and heavily sweetened commercial foods. Such products contain a high percentage of chemical constituents and a low percentage of natural food. In addition, processing of the small amounts of real food in these products is so intensive that most of the nutrients are removed. Chemical additives and processing are used to produce "pseudo" or "phony" food products. Such products look like food, taste like food, but are not really food. They contain few nutrients and are little more than a tasty mixture of chemicals and sweeteners. A good example is many soft drinks—particularly diet beverages. In most, the only natural ingredient is water. Everything else is made in a factory. Second, modern farming techniques have stripped valuable nutrients from the soil, leaving produce that—even though chemically fertilized—is significantly inferior (nutritionally) to that produced one hundred years ago with natural farming techniques.

Another cause of serious nutritional deficiencies is inertia in the conventional medical community. For many years, "experts" have advocated a low-fat, high-grain diet. Such diets have put healthy high-fat foods, like nuts and seeds, in the "eat sparingly" category, and highly processed foods like breads and pastas in the "eat regularly" position. While it is not known how many people actually adhere to the guidelines, statistics on obesity, many cancers, and several other illnesses are still rising. The more forward-looking members of the scientific community have advocated changes in the "classic" food pyramid for at least a decade, but inertia is hard to overcome. This food pyramid, with heavy emphasis on pastas and other refined grain products, and low emphasis on beans, nuts, seeds, and other foods high in plant fats, is possibly the cause of many of the rising statistics for chronic illnesses over the past few decades. It is time for serious reevaluation. Recent changes to the food pyramid have improved it, but, according to many experts, it is still woefully inadequate and overly complicated.

To make matters worse, many nutritionists and other medical professionals continue to insist that vitamin, mineral, and other food supplements are unnecessary and a waste of money. The preponderance of evidence gathered today indicates that many nutrients in our food supply are seriously depleted. A recent article in the *Journal of the American Medical Association* states that vitamin and mineral supplementation is desirable even for those whose diet is good.[20] And, for people that can't (or won't) observe proper dietary habits, supplementation is an absolute necessity!

Alcohol and Tobacco

Alcohol — Until recently, most studies failed to find a link between the use of alcohol and prostate conditions. However, within the past decade, this has changed as more studies have found that the risk of prostate cancer rises with increased alcohol use. Several large studies found that alcohol is a risk factor for developing prostate disease, particularly when consumption is a longtime issue.[21, 22] These studies determined that moderate liquor consumption, defined as three drinks per week to three drinks per day, was associated with a significantly increased risk of prostate cancer, as compared with men who use little to no alcohol. The risks became even more apparent as the number of drinks increased from moderate to heavy (twenty-two or more drinks per week). However, moderate wine and/or beer consumption, from one glass per month to one glass per day, was found to have an insignificant prostate cancer risk. This interesting observation is probably due to the presence of plant-based estrogenic substances (phytoestrogens) in beer and wine that mediate the effects of estrogens produced by the body.[23, 24] It may also account for the fact that alcohol consumption in the form of beer and wine is marginally beneficial.

Excessive alcohol consumption may add to the age-related decrease in testosterone and increased conversion of testosterone to DHT. As blood alcohol levels rise, serum testosterone levels tend to decrease.[25] It is not known if this temporary alcohol-related drop in testosterone levels increases the risk of prostate disease. However, it is probable that high levels of alcohol consumption could cause testosterone levels to be continuously depressed, thus raising the risk of prostate dysfunction. One study in particular noted that men with cirrhosis of the liver due to alcohol consumption had low testosterone levels and increased estrogen levels.[26] A high level of estrogen, unopposed by other androgens or progesterone, is another risk factor for prostate disease. Thus, it is likely that a chronic alcohol-related increase in estrogen coupled with a corresponding decrease in testosterone and other androgens could accelerate the development of prostate disease via the same pathways as advancing age. Several recent studies have made this suggestion. Excessive consumption of alcohol is also known to lead to many other health problems. If you are trying to ameliorate a prostate condition, a good starting point is to put serious limits on the amount of alcohol you consume, particularly in the form of hard liquor.

There has been considerable news in the media about the beneficial effects of wine consumption. Several studies have found consumption of red wine to be protective against certain cancers, including prostate cancer. Some of these studies were financed by the winemaking industry for obvious reasons. Other studies have shown red and purple grape juice to be protective.[27, 28] Any benefits from drinking red wine are likely due to the phytoestrogens in the grapes used to make it. Since alcohol is known to cause problems, I believe a man with prostate problems would be far better off getting his phytoestrogens from grapes instead of wine.

Tobacco — It is well-known that tobacco use (either via smoking or chewing) is a risk factor for serious health conditions, including many cancers. Studies that have examined the relationship between cigarette smoking and prostate disease have not produced consistent links. Some found a loosely associated elevated risk and others have not confirmed any risk. However, recent studies suggest a link between heavy smoking and the occurrence of fatal prostate cancer, particularly when smoking continues into late life.[29, 30, 31] This may simply be because the general health of smokers is poorer than nonsmokers. Also of significance is that current cigarette smokers were found to have significantly higher levels of androstenedione, estrone, and estradiol as compared to nonsmokers.[32] Again, high levels of estrogens have been positively linked to many prostate and breast disorders, including cancer. Virtually all of the studies agree that the risk increases proportionally with the number of years smoking and with the number of cigarettes smoked per day.[33] The studies also agree that quitting reduces risk, and the risk proportionally decreases with the number of years passed since quitting.

Thus, while no evidence for an association between smoking and prostate disease was found as little as a decade ago, the current data presents overwhelming evidence that smoking is detrimental to one's overall health in general, and that it is also a strong risk factor in developing aggressive, and possibly fatal, prostate cancer.[34] If you are trying to resolve a prostate problem, smoking is certainly not in your favor.

Pesticides and Other Environmental Issues

An interesting note is that a higher risk of prostate disease is found in smokers that are also exposed to cadmium. Cadmium is a trace element that occurs in varying concentration in cigarette smoke. It is also found in alkaline batteries, industries where electroplating and welding occurs, and several other industries. Studies appear to have found a link between exposure to cadmium and the development of various cancers, including prostate and breast cancer.[35] With prostate cancer, the risk was most apparent for aggressive tumors.[36] Most of the studies base this on the hypothesis that cadmium reduces the body's ability to absorb zinc, a necessary element for many cellular processes, and an element of particular importance to the prostate. (See zinc in Chapter Seven.)

Another risk factor is exposure to environmental pesticides. Several studies have found a significantly higher risk among farm workers and licensed pesticide applicators.[37, 38] Interestingly, cancers that are primarily associated with estrogen disrupters were found in male, but not female, pesticide applicators. The workers risk appeared to be increased with specific chemicals, primarily those in the family of organophosphate pesticides like lindane and heptachlor, fumigants like methyl bromide, or triazine herbicides. Significant increases in the risk of developing prostate disease were linked to the use of chlorinated pesticides.[39] One study looked at leisure-time exposure. It found an increased risk for men whose work or leisure activities consistently exposed them to the fumes or bodily absorption of certain chemicals.[40] Activities most implicated were those that resulted in exposure to chemicals used in painting, stripping, or varnishing furniture, exposure to metal dusts, and exposure to lubricating oils or greases. Also, repeated exposure to home or garden pesticide sprays was noted as an increased risk factor. In all studies, risk was directly related to amounts of exposure.

Vasectomy

Another factor that affects hormone balance is the male sterilization procedure, vasectomy. In this procedure the vas deferens tubes are cut, eliminating the path sperm take from the testicles to the prostate.* A vasectomy is a minor surgical procedure, generally taking about 20-30 minutes. It is usually performed in a doctor's office with local anesthesia.

In the 1970s, vasectomy became a popular birth control method. Since then, several medical reports linked it to prostate cancer, and roughly an equal number of studies found no association. The more recent reports have not found any statistically significant link, but the issue remains controversial.[41, 42, 43, 44, 45, 46] In the years following a vasectomy, there is a small but measurable increase in total testosterone, but no corresponding increase in free (or unbound) testosterone. In fact, free testosterone tends to decrease after a vasectomy. Thus, more circulating (bound) testosterone may also mean more of it is being converted to DHT. Since all hormones—and particularly the sex hormones—are interdependent, it is entirely possible that this small increase in testosterone represents only the tip of the iceberg. While research has not conclusively linked prostate cancer and vasectomy, it is interesting to note the paragraph quoted below from one study,

> . . . a higher ratio of DHT to testosterone was found among vasectomized control subjects than among nonvasectomized control subjects. The findings do not support previous reports of increased prostate cancer risk associated with vasectomy. However, the altered endocrine profiles of vasectomized control subjects warrant further evaluation in longitudinal studies. . . .[47]

Increased DHT to testosterone ratio appears to be linked to prostate disease, including cancer. While the authors of this report did not find statistically significant evidence that supports additional prostate cancer risk, they note that vasectomized subjects have *altered endocrine profiles*, and that further evaluation is warranted. Other studies have noted a trend towards increased risk of

---

*The vas deferens are the tubes that carry the sperm cells from the testicles to the ejaculatory ducts. Cutting them results in male sterilization.

prostate cancer as the number of years from the surgical vasectomy increased. Again, this trend was not statistically significant.

The bottom line is that the so-called "harmless" vasectomy, while not specifically linked to the development of prostate cancer, has, according to almost all of the studies, side effects on a man's hormonal profile. These effects appear to become more pronounced with the passage of time and might be linked to problems like erectile dysfunction and loss of libido. Of course, this is of little comfort for a man who had a vasectomy in his thirties and is now facing prostate problems in his fifties, sixties, or seventies!

Vasectomy works quite well for the purposes of contraception. However, there are other methods of contraception that also work. A young man considering the procedure should weigh the potential effects of hormone imbalances it may cause at some future date. If you have already had a vasectomy, you should monitor your free hormone levels regularly, and maintain their balance via herbal supplementation and natural hormone replacement. Chapters nine and ten explain how to do this.

Summary

There are many factors that affect the body's hormone balance. Aging, lifestyle, and environmental pollutants all influence human hormone levels. To some extent, these imbalances are controllable. Proper herbal and nutritional support can help restore age-related hormone imbalances. Changes in diet and lifestyle can reduce environmental influences. And, supplementing with bio-identical hormones can help restore normal balance.

In this chapter, we have examined some factors that affect hormone balance. Achieving a state of relative balance between male (androgen) and the female (estrogen) hormones is critical towards maintaining prostate health. In Part II of this book, we examine many ways to restore this balance.

Chapter Five

Health Conditions and Erectile Dysfunction

In the preceding chapters, we examined hormone imbalances as they relate to prostate dysfunction. In this chapter, we review the mechanism of an erection and some common health conditions that typically coexist in men with erectile dysfunction.

Disruption of hormone levels, particularly when testosterone levels are low, can result in poor sexual function and loss of libido. However, while low testosterone levels can affect erectile performance, more often the problem is a side effect of other health conditions. Impotence (erectile dysfunction) is often caused by seemingly unrelated health conditions or is a side effect of medical treatment.* Many medications, especially antidepressants, can cause or exacerbate it. Thus, an unwary man can easily become trapped in a vicious cycle. His low testosterone levels can cause depression as well as a decrease in libido. If his depression is treated with antidepressants, his libido may decrease even more, and he may experience medication-related erectile dysfunction, further increasing his depression and compounding his problems. [1, 2, 3, 4, 5, 6]

Most men have few problems with erectile dysfunction in their youth and expect such youthful vigor to continue forever. However, as the years advance, the health and vitality of the body deteriorates, and the level of sexual vigor drops accordingly. Unfortunately, many men suffering from erectile dysfunction or

---

* In this book, I use the terms "impotence," "erectile dysfunction," and "ED" interchangeably.

loss of libido, cannot (or will not) admit to a connection between their overall health and their sexual problems. Fortunately, most such problems can be corrected.[7]

Many cases of erectile dysfunction are due to impaired blood circulation resulting from an underlying health condition. All body organs and tissues depend on circulating blood to provide necessary nutrients and remove waste products. An organ lacking good blood circulation cannot maintain peak health. The prostate is no exception. It is well supplied with blood vessels and capillaries, and dependent on them to maintain its function.* The overall health of the prostate and the nerve bundles that surround it are crucial to sexual performance and satisfaction.

The penis is also dependent on good blood circulation. Like the prostate, it needs an ample blood supply for nourishment. However, aside from general tissue health, the penis requires unimpeded blood circulation to produce an erection for sexual activity. Thus, while some cases of erectile dysfunction are related to hormone imbalances, the problem is more often a direct result of poor health or vascular insufficiency.† Any health condition, medication, or physical injury that impedes blood circulation in a man often results in some degree of prostate problems or erectile dysfunction. Many chronic conditions are also a result of decreased blood flow in the body. Thus, erectile dysfunction can be the first symptom of a compromised vascular system, and is often an early symptom of other cardiovascular problems.[8]

Mechanism of an Erection

A man's erection is a complex event that is dependent on many factors. Among them are a proper emotional setting, a good mental attitude, proper nervous system action, correct hormone levels, and an

---

* Capillaries are minute, hair-like blood vessels.

† Vascular insufficiency is a more precise term for impaired blood circulation.

adequate supply of blood to the genitals. All of these items are, to a large extent, dependent on the overall health and vitality of the body. In the past, the belief was that erectile dysfunction was primarily a psychological problem. However, it is now well accepted that most impotence is a direct result of vascular problems. Of course, the foregoing statement ignores impotence caused by medications, physical deformity, or physical trauma. For successful sexual activity, the penis must become rigid enough to allow vaginal penetration, and must remain in a rigid state long enough for intercourse to be completed. This is accomplished by a superb, but remarkably simple plumbing design that is almost entirely dependent on blood flow as shown in the Figure 1 below.

The penis contains two major chambers called *corpora cavernosa (penis)*, and a smaller inner chamber called *corpora cavernosa (urethra) or corpora spongiosa*. The larger chambers run the entire length of the penis on each side and the smaller one runs down the middle and expands at the end to form the organ's head. (See Figure 1.) All three chambers consist of highly expandable sponge-like tissue, and it is the filling of this tissue with blood that produces the male erection.

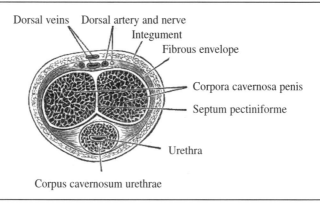

FIGURE 1. Cross section of the human penis*

* Source: Anatomy of the Human Body, 1918, Henry Gray (1825-1861), Figure 1155.

When a man becomes aroused, a complex interaction of various hormones, nerve signals, and chemical processes begin that initiate action in the blood vessels and muscles of the penis. Its blood vessels start to dilate, allowing more blood to flow into the three chambers, and it begins to expand. At the same time, muscles at the base of the penis restrict blood flowing back to the body. Thus, more blood is inbound than outbound. When fully erect, a man's penis contains between six and eight times as much blood as when it is not erect. It is not difficult to see how a blockage in the arteries that feed the penile chambers, or a general insufficiency in blood flow, can cause problems with erections.*

Underlying Health Problems

There are many health conditions that contribute to vascular problems, and any one of them can cause or exacerbate erectile dysfunction. For many years, impotence was thought to be a side effect or complication of other vascular problems like diabetes, cardiovascular disease, high blood pressure, high cholesterol or high triglyceride levels.† However, it is more likely that impotence is the earliest indicator of impaired circulation problems from one of the above conditions. Thus, by resolving problems with erectile dysfunction early and naturally, one may also be preventing or ameliorating other cardiovascular problems. [9, 10, 11]

Several studies have found erectile dysfunction to be prevalent among men with high total cholesterol and low HDL/LDL ratios. High cholesterol and triglyceride levels are well-known as strong risk factors for numerous cardiovascular problems.[12] Reducing their levels can help correct erectile dysfunction while

---

* A more detailed discussion of the erection mechanism can be found in the book *The Testosterone Syndrome* (see the bibliography). Also see—"Chemicals Involved in an Erection"—in Chapter Nine.

* Triglycerides are fatty acids in the blood. High levels often occur with high cholesterol levels.

also lowering the risk of other problems.[13] These elevated levels can be reduced with prescription medication or herbal remedies. However, since they usually result from a poor diet and lack of exercise, lifestyle and dietary changes are significantly more effective and should be the first choice. Often, high cholesterol and triglyceride levels are accompanied by or result in high blood pressure (hypertension), hardening of the arteries (arteriosclerosis), or arteries clogged by cholesterol deposits (atherosclerosis). These conditions all inhibit blood flow in the body, and can be grouped under the general term of vascular or cardiovascular dysfunction.

Diabetes can also cause serious problems. It exacerbates erectile dysfunction by making blood vessels less elastic. Such blood vessels cannot dilate fully and thus restrict blood flow during an erection. Diabetes also deteriorates nerve viability, thus decreasing the sensitivity of the penis. Both effects are magnified when the condition has been present or poorly controlled for many years. A side effect of long-term uncontrolled diabetes is nearly always severe impotence. Diabetes also has profound effects on the endocrine system and thus on hormone levels. A recent study in *The Journal of Clinical Endocrinology and Metabolism* measured testosterone levels of 103 men with type-2 diabetes and found that 33 percent of them had low free testosterone levels.[14] The median age of these men was 54.7 years. In this study, the men seemed to have lowered levels of the pituitary hormones that control testosterone production. This is interesting because it suggests that diabetes lowers free testosterone levels by a process unrelated to aging. Essentially, this means that age-related declines in testosterone levels are magnified in the presence of diabetes. This is another good reason for any diabetic to monitor his condition carefully and keep it under control.

Similarly, the blockage of veins and arteries due to arteriosclerosis and atherosclerosis can cause or exacerbate impotence by physically diminishing blood flow to the penis. Hypertension is frequently the result of clogged arteries from either condition. When the body's circulation system is clogged with deposits, the heart must pump harder to move blood around the body, thus raising blood pressure. And even though the heart is pumping harder, blood flow is still diminished from normal.

The obvious conclusion is that conditions that impair blood flow throughout the body affect all organs, including the prostate and the penis. As mentioned before, when the blood supply to any organ in the body is diminished, the health of the organ deteriorates. And when blood flow to penile arteries is impeded, erectile dysfunction is inevitable.

Erectile dysfunction can be quite debilitating to a sexually active man and his partner. It is often the first symptom of a more serious problem—one of clogged arteries and poor blood circulation. Many studies have confirmed this, including a recent article published in the *Journal of the American Medical Association* (JAMA).[15] According to its authors, data from this large study (9,457 men) provides evidence of a strong association between erectile dysfunction and subsequent development of cardiovascular problems. The simple truth is that when blood circulation is poor in one area of the body—the penile arteries—it is very likely deficient in many other parts of the body as well, including arteries that supply the heart (and the brain).

Viagra® and Its Cousins

Studies have shown that more than half the male population over the age of fifty suffers from ED to some degree. Thus, it is a significant problem for the aging male. Many men, no doubt influenced by constant bombardment of ED drug advertisements, view it as a simple problem that can (or should) be quickly remedied with a prescription drug. Unfortunately, some of their overworked doctors simply do not take the time to evaluate all their risk factors before reaching for a prescription pad.

While treating ED with medication typically results in a happy patient, it does little to correct underlying circulation problems which are then allowed to progress unchecked. Prescribing an ED drug without dealing with such underlying vascular issues is blindly treating a symptom while ignoring the problem. Eventually, the erectile dysfunction may be of little concern when a man begins to suffer from serious vascular problems such as angina, a coronary event, or a stroke. Remember that "ignorance is bliss" smile we talked about earlier? It fades quickly after a heart attack!

As I mentioned in the introduction, I was lucky to have suffered from erectile dysfunction back in the days before Viagra® (Sildenafil citrate), Cialis® (Tadalafil), and Levitra® (Vardenafil). Back then, I had no choice but to use vitamins, herbs, and lifestyle changes if I wanted to regain some semblance of my former sexual ability. Today, a man doesn't have to work that hard. A quick trip to the doctor will usually result in a prescription for one of the three, and in most cases, the *symptoms* of impotence will be resolved. Any man who feels this is the best course of action is fooling himself in a big way!

ED drugs are not risk-free. A recent report in the *Journal of Neuro-Ophthalmology* found seven men who, after taking Viagra, had typical features of a condition known as nonarteritic ischemic optic neuropathy (NAION).[16] This condition appears to cause damage to the retina of the eye when blood flow to the retina or optic nerve is cut off—essentially producing a stroke in the eye. The result is sudden vision loss, permanent injury to the nerve, and in some cases, permanent blindness. The report went on to say that all of the affected individuals had pre-existing conditions like hypertension, diabetes, or elevated cholesterol or lipid levels and concluded that Viagra may induce NAION in individuals with this typical risk profile. Considering that many men that need Viagra have a similar risk profile, it is obvious that Viagra can increase the risk of eye-related problems. Of course, this caused quite a stir in the media and was followed by statements from Viagra's manufacturer (Pfizer) insisting on its safety. According to an article in the *San Francisco Chronicle* on July 1, 2005, more than 800 cases of eye problems were reported to the FDA after using Viagra. Of these cases, more than 100 resulted in partial or total blindness.* On July

---

* While this discussion refers specifically to Viagra, the other impotence drugs could cause similar problems.

8, 2005, the government ordered warnings to be put on the labels of the three FDA approved erectile dysfunction drugs while it continues to investigate. The news that Viagra and other anti-impotence drugs may have effects on vision is not new. A paper from the *American Academy of Ophthalmology* in November of 2003 also mentioned such effects, as did some earlier studies.[17] Carefully worded warnings are also in the literature that comes with the drug. Looking at this evidence, one can only conclude that if you are willing to take Viagra or its analogs to improve sexual function, you are also willing to risk your eyesight. To this writer, even though the risk is very low, this is not always an acceptable trade-off.

Sometimes side effects of a drug can take years to surface. For example, Viagra, which has been on the market for almost a decade, was recently shown to exacerbate respiratory problems in men with sleep apnea, a condition where a sleeping person repeatedly stops breathing.[18]

In addition to the other problems detailed above, both Viagra and Levitra have been associated with epileptic seizures. A recent paper published in the *British Medical Journal* reported two cases of epileptic seizures after taking Viagra. Both men were relatively young, (aged 63 and 54) and had no previous history of epilepsy or other neurological conditions. Four similar cases were also reported to the Viagra's manufacturer during clinical trials, but at that time, no correlation was found to the seizures.[19] More recently, animal tests using Viagra have shown a convulsion-inducing effect. This effect increased when Viagra was combined with L-Arginine, an essential amino acid often used to enhance nitric oxide levels in men with erectile dysfunction.[20] (See Chapter Nine.) In addition, Levitra, which was approved by the FDA in August of 2003 (Viagra was introduced in 1998), has also had recent reports linking it to epileptic seizures in otherwise healthy men.[21, 22]

As I wrote earlier in this chapter, impotence has several causes, the most common being impaired blood circulation to penile arteries or hormone imbalances. Drugs cause a temporary increase in blood flow, resulting in a firmer erection. However, they do not clear clogged arteries nor do they correct hormone levels. While they provide effective short-term relief from symptoms, they do little to rectify any underlying conditions. A permanent solution for erectile dysfunction is best achieved by addressing the problem at its source through lifestyle changes and improvement of overall health.

If you are willing to accept the risks, you can use an ED drug to temporarily alleviate the immediate problem. However, this should be considered only as a temporary solution. In that case, discuss the temporary use of Cialis with your doctor. The FDA approved Cialis in November 2003. It has a profile that is less likely to cause disturbances with the retina of the eye, and at the time of this writing, I could not find any reports of it causing other problems.[23] Impotence can be a major annoyance to any man. But treating its source is far more conducive to good health than putting a "band-aid" on it with an ED drug. A heart attack or a stroke from untreated circulation problems, or hormone related prostate cancer, as well as blindness or epileptic seizures are far more threatening.

Summary of Part I

In Part I we have taken a detailed, albeit simplified, look at some body functions, that when disrupted, can cause prostate or sexual dysfunction. Chief among these are imbalances in the sex steroid hormones and vascular problems. We have looked at the probable causes of hormone imbalances, and, in particular, examined the effects of aging and environmental estrogen mimics (pseudoestrogens or xenoestrogens) on hormone balance. This chapter concludes Part I with a discussion of some of the health conditions that accompany erectile dysfunction. I have chosen to discuss ED separately in both parts of this book for several reasons, not the least of which is that it is a condition that effects most men over fifty. Also, it is my firm belief that erectile dysfunction is a precursor to more serious problems, and that correcting it can and should be done naturally, with minimum use of drugs.

As we move towards the second part of this book, I hope the information provided in Part I will help you to better understand which natural techniques in Part II are best for you. Now that we have looked at some of the causes of these problems, it is time to look at some natural ways to prevent or reverse them. Chapters Six through Nine show you how to do this by changing your environment, avoiding agents that trigger problems, getting proper nutrition, supplementing with appropriate vitamins, minerals, and herbal agents, and using natural hormones to rebalance those that have gone astray. Chapter Ten shows you many specific ways you can correct erectile dysfunction problems naturally, and finally, Chapter Eleven shows you how to create a supplementation plan that fits your individual needs.

PART II

NATURAL WAYS TO STRENGTHEN YOUR PROSTATE

Chapter Six

Let There Be Light

It is evident from research that prostate dysfunction is caused by a combination of factors: some nutritional, some lifestyle, and some as side effects of other clinical conditions. In addition there is much overlap between items that are typically called lifestyle factors and those that are deemed nutritional. For example, eating habits can be considered to span both the lifestyle and nutritional category. Also, sunlight striking bare skin is the most efficient way for the body to get vitamin D, an item that is critically important for the prevention of prostate disease. Production of vitamin D (a nutrient) is a direct result of exposure to sunlight (a lifestyle issue). Since vitamin D controls so many interrelated body processes, some researchers suggest it should be called a hormone. Several books have called it the "sunshine hormone."

For many years, experts have advised people to avoid all sun exposure. The reasoning is that exposing bare skin to the sun raises the risk of developing skin cancer. Excessive sun exposure and frequent severe sunburns, particularly during childhood, have been linked to an increased risk of developing melanoma, the most severe and life-threatening form of skin cancer. But this link is not proven. The national cancer institute website, says: "There is inadequate evidence to determine whether the avoidance of sunburns alters the incidence of cutaneous melanoma."

On the other hand solid evidence continues to mount that a lack of sun exposure contributes significantly to the development of other cancers. While this appears to be contradictory, it is not. Frequent exposure to the sun for short periods, without burning, does not substantially increase the risk of skin cancer. Such exposure is actually protective against the development of many chronic diseases and cancers and is specifically relevant to prostate cancer.[1, 2]

Sunlight, Vitamin D and Prostate Cancer

Resistance to change often inhibits progress. Many of us have indeed heeded the warnings, avoided sun exposure, and diligently used sunblocking agents. However, the incidence of many cancers continues to rise. Since the early part of the last century, research has suggested that sunlight helps lower the risk of cancer. Geographical studies show an association between living at higher latitudes and increased cancer risk. However, the prevailing wisdom has been to avoid sun exposure due to the risk of some skin cancers. This long-term purveyance of the idea that *any* exposure to the sun increases the risk of skin cancer has induced an unreasonable fear of the sun in many people. Such unfounded fears have led to an inordinate avoidance of sun exposure and a consequential deficiency of vitamin D.

The primary way the human body gets vitamin D is from the sun. Human beings have a built-in mechanism for obtaining vitamin D through the action of sunlight on their exposed skin. Insufficient sun exposure results in vitamin D deficiency. Many experts estimate that more than 80 percent of the U.S. population is severely deficient in vitamin D, especially during the winter months. The effect of this deficiency on the prostate and other organs in the body is profound.[3, 4, 5] Recent studies have concluded that vitamin D deficiency is a significant risk factor for the development of many diseases, including breast and prostate cancer.[6, 7, 8] The authors of one study wrote:

> Confirming that vitamin D levels indeed account for the associations we observed is critical because current health recommendations typically discourage high intake of vitamin

D and high levels of sun exposure, at least without use of sunscreen, which effectively blocks vitamin D production.[9]

Tomasz Beer, M.D., an oncologist, and others have research currently under way using a form of high dose vitamin D (known as DN-101) intravenously in an attempt to slow the progress of existing prostate cancer.[10] As of this writing, this research is ongoing and has not yet been proven, but it underscores the importance the scientific community is placing on vitamin D and its relationship to cancer.

In many studies, vitamin D supplementation has been shown to improve the outcome for people with cardiovascular problems, arthritis, depression, diabetes, hypertension, kidney problems, cancer, and other chronic conditions.[11, 12, 13, 14, 15, 16]

Few foods contain significant amounts of vitamin D, and unfortunately, those that do are typically not consumed in sufficient quantity by much of the population. Obtaining sufficient vitamin D solely from food is difficult, if not impossible, particularly in light of the nutrient-poor fast foods many people consume. In addition, aging contributes to deficiencies in older individuals by reducing the body's ability to synthesize vitamin D from sunlight.[17]

Regarding sun exposure—all myths are encapsulated in a kernel of truth. There is truth in the statement that sunlight can be harmful. Excessive exposure to the sun can damage human skin. Multiple severe sunburns cause skin damage. Damaged skin is subject to disease, the most serious of which is skin cancer. While short intervals of sun exposure are essential, one should never allow the skin to be damaged by burning. It is interesting to note that many older studies that linked skin cancer to sun exposure were done using fair-skinned people. Fair skin is much more susceptible to sun damage than darker skin. During the summer months, ten to fifteen minutes of exposure, two to three times per week, is sufficient to produce adequate vitamin D levels in most people with light skin. Darker skinned people need more.

A wealth of evidence indicates that prostate problems and vitamin D deficiency are linked.[18] Several studies have shown that black men living in Africa, have much lower rates of prostate cancer than black men living in America.[19, 20, 21] In the past, researchers theorized that this was due to the adaptation of a westernized diet. However, dark skin absorbs less sunlight and thus produces less vitamin D than fair skin for the same relative sun exposure. Historically, black men lived in tropical areas where considerable sun exposure was inevitable. Their skin pigmentation protected them from *excessive* exposure. On migrating to northern areas, this built-in genetic protection becomes a liability. Due to the limited strength and duration of sunlight in northern climates, particularly in the winter months, black men (and woman) are unable to produce the minimum amount of vitamin D needed by their bodies. Fair-skinned people living in northern climates have similar deficiencies, albeit to a lesser degree.

A recent study of overall sun exposure versus skin pigmentation concluded that susceptibility to prostate cancer is in part determined by the extent of exposure to the sun, and that skin pigmentation (or the ability for the skin to tan) mediated the sun's overall effect.[22] In other words, a suntan—but not a sunburn—is healthy. Natural health practitioners have been saying this for years. This same study indicated that cumulative exposure to sunlight was less in the group of men with prostate cancer than those with BPH, or in other words the men who had more lifetime sun exposure had less prostate cancer!

During winter months in the United States, it is virtually impossible to get sufficient sunlight to forestall a vitamin D deficiency, even for those with fair skin. The only real exception to this is for people who live in southern Florida, southern Texas, or Hawaii. Nearly everyone living north of these areas is subject to a vitamin D deficiency for the greater part of the year. Several studies have examined the geographical incidence of prostate cancer. Virtually all of them found an increased incidence of prostate cancer in northern areas subject to long winters with little sunlight. The same was true of breast and colon cancers. This correlates directly with levels of ultraviolet radiation from the sun and associated vitamin D production by the skin.[23, 24, 25, 26, 27, 28]

Exposure to sunlight easily corrects vitamin D deficiencies. However, when sunlight is minimal, supplementation with vitamin D is appropriate. It is important that such supplementation should be prudent. One study noted in increase in prostate problems with excessive supplementation of vitamin D.[29] The current recommended daily allowance (RDA) of vitamin D is 200 IU for those under fifty, 400 IU from fifty to seventy, and 600 IU for adults over seventy. However, this may be inadequate, especially for older adults. A recent review of several studies noted that the concentrations of vitamin D needed to maintain good health could not be reached with the currently recommended RDAs. The authors of the review suggest that raising the RDA of vitamin D for all adults to at least 1000 IU will help prevent many serious chronic conditions, particularly in older adults.[30] The maximum daily intake of Vitamin D known to be safe is currently 2000 IU.

Recent studies have now demonstrated that avoidance of the sun and the use of sunscreens is *not* the best strategy for reducing the overall incidence of cancer, particularly prostate cancer. Moderate exposure to the sun—rather than total avoidance—is much more reasonable and effective.

Vitamin D and Calcium

Vitamin D has many roles in the body. The classical one is as a mediator of calcium absorption. The ability of the body to utilize calcium is greatly impaired in the presence of a vitamin D deficiency. Studies have linked vitamin D deficiency to various bone and muscle defects, including osteoporosis.[31] In addition, evidence indicates that simultaneous supplementation with both vitamin D and calcium reduced the risk of colorectal cancer significantly.[32] However, as with vitamin D, excess calcium intake is controversial. In one study, a total calcium intake (from diet and supplements) greater than 2000mg/day was associated with modestly increased risk of prostate cancer.[33]

As with most nutrients, vitamin D appears to work synergistically with other elements. In addition to its important role in balancing the body's calcium levels, vitamin D is an important modulator of growth and cell differentiation in both breast and prostate tissue, and is thus protective against cancer development and progression.[34, 35, 36, 37, 38] Differentiation is the process by which dividing cells take on the characteristics of the tissue or organ they are part of. Cells that do not differentiate properly are abnormal and usually destroyed by the body or self-destruct on their own (a process called apoptosis). Abnormal, undifferentiated cells that are not destroyed eventually result in the uncontrolled growth of cancer.

From the many studies on calcium and vitamin D, it is obvious that there is a synergistic relationship between them and other nutrients, and that maintaining optimal levels of vitamin D can reduce the risk of many illnesses, including those of the prostate.

Measuring Vitamin D Levels

The best way to keep your vitamin D levels within the correct range is to have your levels measured. A naturopathic or nutritionally-oriented medical doctor can do this for you easily. The test is called 25(OH)D or 25-hydroxyvitaminD. Vitamin D blood levels have a relatively narrow range and excessive amounts can be harmful. Before doing the test or supplementing, I suggest you learn more about optimal vitamin D levels. For more information, I suggest Dr. Joseph Mercola's website as a starting point. (See the appendix.) Other sites specifically devoted to Vitamin D are in the appendix, and there are some books listed in the bibliography.

People who live in northern areas can supplement during the winter months, or when they cannot get out into the sun regularly. Most over-the-counter multivitamins sold today contain 200 to 400 International Units (IU) of Vitamin D. The best sources are made from fish oil. During the summer months, a multivitamin plus some sun exposure is more than adequate. During winter months, an additional 400 to 600 IU can be taken safely in most of the U.S.[39]

Vitamin D and Your Immune System

In the beginning of this chapter, we discussed the importance of sun exposure to produce vitamin D for general health and prevention of prostate problems. Vitamin D also plays a crucial role in stimulating the immune system and reducing inflammation caused by conditions such as rheumatoid arthritis.[40, 41] Inflammation is also linked to many other chronic conditions including cardiovascular disease (CVD). As explained in Chapter 5, CVD is a condition often linked to prostate and sexual problems. Vitamin D is a critical nutrient vital to maintaining a strong immune system.

A Note of Caution

If your doctor checks your vitamin D levels and finds them deficient, you may be put on a prescription vitamin D medication. As a supplement, Vitamin D comes in two forms: ergocalciferol (vitamin D2) and cholecalciferol (vitamin D3). Vitamin D3 is the natural form, identical to that produced by your body when it is exposed to sunshine. Most prescription vitamin D is the synthetic form. Recent studies have shown it to be considerably less effective. Make sure you are only prescribed vitamin D as D3 (cholecalciferol).[42]

Summary

Unfortunately, there are many professionals who still espouse the idea that humans evolved similar to subterranean insects like termites, and thus they should not be exposed to sunlight in any way. Nothing is further from the truth. Human beings evolved naked, in tropical climates, without access to sun-blocking chemicals.* We

---

*It is beyond the scope of this book to discuss the pros and cons of using sunblocking preparations. However, it is interesting to note that in the course of my research I came across several recent reports—published in prestigious medical journals— that suggest the increasing use of sunblocking preparations may be linked to the rising incidence of melanoma, the most deadly form of skin cancer.

are programmed to get our vitamin D from direct exposure to sunlight, and nothing can change this! Recent reports have indicated that while avoidance of the sun may reduce the risk of certain skin cancers, most skin cancers are rather inconsequential. However, vitamin D deficiency induced by sun avoidance may significantly increase the risk of developing potentially more serious cancers, like prostate cancer. A recent study looking at the period from 1986 to 2001 concluded that the rising incidence of melanoma (the most serious and often fatal skin cancer) is not due to an actual increase in the disease, but is rather due to increased diagnostic scrutiny for the condition. The report also noted that mortality due to this condition was stable over the study period, and the incidence of other chronic illnesses, including many cancers, increased.[43] According to this report, avoiding sun exposure has had little effect on the incidence of the most serious skin cancer and may possibly increase the incidence of other conditions.

Adequate exposure of bare skin to sunlight is essential for good health. More specifically, adequate vitamin D levels resulting from exposure to sunlight, supplementation, or both are essential for the prevention of prostate problems—specifically prostate cancer.

Chapter Seven

The Basics of Prostate (and General) Health

To keep your prostate healthy, it is important to supply it with the proper balance of nutrients. From these nutrients, the body manufactures hormones to control the actions of its organs. To do this, it needs high quality fuel. The food we eat contains vitamins, minerals, enzymes, and other substances that comprise this fuel. Collectively, these are called nutrients or micronutrients.* When it comes to fuel, many of us treat our automobiles better than our bodies. If you want your car to perform well, you give it high quality fuel. The same applies to your body. This chapter is about the special nutrients that fuel healthy prostate action.

It can be said that nutrient deficiencies are at the root of many chronic conditions. Unfortunately, it is a formidable (and often impossible) task to determine nutrient deficiencies that cause disease with absolute certainty since many disorders are the result of a multitude of factors. Prostate dysfunction is known to be multifactorial. No specific nutrient deficiencies have proven to be a definitive cause of prostate disease. However, there is much evidence that links hormone imbalances to prostate and sexual problems. What is unknown is all of the mechanisms that cause such imbalances. Some are obvious while others are subtle. Research suggests that certain nutritional deficiencies are linked to the development of disease.

---

*Micronutrients are items (typically minerals) that are essential for good health in extremely small amounts.

For decades health experts have resisted recommending vitamin and mineral supplements—insisting instead that all needed nutrients can be obtained from a proper diet. Within the recent past, this damaging paradigm has finally been abandoned. A recent article in the *Journal of the American Medical Association* confirmed that supplemental vitamins and minerals can help prevent chronic diseases.[1] This is a significant milestone. The report concluded that intake levels of several vitamins could be well above levels classically defined for deficiency levels, and still be suboptimal, and pose a risk for several chronic diseases, particularly in the elderly.

> … suboptimal intake of some vitamins, above levels causing classic vitamin deficiency, is a risk factor for chronic diseases and common in the general population, especially the elderly. Suboptimal folic acid levels, along with suboptimal levels of vitamins B_6 and B_{12}, are a risk factor for cardiovascular disease, neural tube defects, and colon and breast cancer; low levels of vitamin D contribute to osteopenia and fractures; and low levels of the antioxidant vitamins (vitamins A, E, and C) may increase risk for several chronic diseases.[1]

It goes on to say that most people do not consume an optimal amount of vitamins through their diet alone. Elderly or chronically ill adults or those with malabsorption problems may be at increased risk of severe deficiencies, particularly of B vitamins. Deficiencies of folate and vitamins B_6 and B_{12} are associated with heart disease, and deficiencies of vitamin E, selenium, and lycopene can increase the risk of prostate disease. The obvious conclusion is that an adequate intake of vitamins, minerals, and other nutrients from food and supplements is essential for good health.

The article also discusses increased risk with suboptimal levels of various vitamins. But what exactly is suboptimal? We know, for example, that vitamin C deficiencies cause scurvy, a disease that is quite rare in today's world. Once this fact was known a daily recommended dietary allowance (RDA) of vitamin C was established that would prevent scurvy. RDAs for other vitamins and minerals were also established based on the amount needed to prevent diseases of deficiency. Unfortunately, the RDA for most vitamins and minerals continues to be based on the prevention of deficiency diseases, rather than on enhancing health or prevention of chronic illness.

Most experts agree that the RDAs are far too low for the prevention of chronic diseases though there is much disagreement on what the optimum levels of various nutrients are. Many natural health professionals recommend increased intake of nutrients far in excess of their RDA, especially when the body is abnormally stressed. In most cases, such levels are safe. However, there are some nutrients (like vitamin A) that can become toxic at high doses.

There are many vitamins and minerals that are necessary for the maintenance of life. Some of these are micronutrients where the body needs a very small amount, while others are macronutrients where much larger quantities are needed. Supplements of micronutrients are typically measured in micrograms (mcg) and macronutrients in milligrams (mg.).* Generally, a balanced diet that incorporates vegetables, fruits and a good multivitamin will provide the nutrients for general health.† One important criterion in selecting a multivitamin is to be aware that a day's supply of many needed macronutrients (like calcium) often cannot fit into a small capsule. Thus, many "one-a-day" type vitamin tablets are limited in value. Most quality multivitamins require three to six capsules per day to reach optimal nutrient quantities. It is also important to understand that vitamin supplements are just—*supplements*. You cannot expect to maintain good health by taking vitamins and eating poorly. Vitamin and other food supplements are not substitutes for good dietary and lifestyle habits.

It is impossible to discuss all of the vitamins, minerals and other nutrients vital to human health without writing several thousand pages. Thus, I have limited this book to items where significant

---

* A microgram is one-millionth of a gram. A milligram is one-thousandth of a gram.

† In Chapter Eleven I have provided a typical list of ingredients for a good multivitamin.

research has determined a proven value in maintaining prostate health, general health, or ameliorating prostate problems. In this chapter, we cover the vitamins, minerals, and specific foods that are known to help with prostate dysfunction. In the next chapter, we describe some helpful herbs. Obviously, there are many other nutrients that are helpful towards building general health that are not in this chapter or the next. In Chapter Eleven, I have provided a general supplement plan you can customize for your own situation.

Free Radicals and Antioxidants

An automobile engine burns fuel (gasoline), mixed with air (oxygen) to produce energy. The energy produced is then transferred to the wheels allowing for movement. As the engine burns gasoline, waste products like carbon monoxide and other chemicals are produced and removed via an exhaust system. Similarly, a human body burns fuel (food) with air (oxygen) to generate energy needed for daily life and in the process produces waste products. Of course this is a simple analogy. Both processes are far more complicated, but the overall idea is the same. Fuel is burned to generate energy, which results in production of waste products. In the human body energy production takes place within the body's cells and is called oxidation or metabolism.

Free radicals are waste products from the body's normal metabolism, just as exhaust gases are a normal result of operating a motor vehicle. Like automotive exhaust fumes, free radicals are highly reactive and can be quite destructive. In the body they cause damage to cells if they are not neutralized or removed quickly. Such damage is typically called "oxidative stress" and is believed to be a primary cause of chronic deterioration. For example, it is believed that cardiovascular disease is the result of chronic inflammation of arteries leading to the heart due to oxidative damage from free radicals.

A healthy body neutralizes free radicals into harmless compounds before they do significant damage. Neutralization takes place with the aid of compounds called antioxidants, which quickly combine with free radicals to render them harmless. Antioxidants are chemical compounds that neutralize free radicals and protect the body's cells against the potentially harmful effects of oxidation.

Antioxidants are present in virtually all foods, many supplements, and herbs. They are abundant in a healthy body. An ample supply ensures that the waste products of cellular metabolism are disposed of efficiently. Using the automotive analogy, our automobile would not run well if its exhaust was blocked. In a similar manner, our bodies will not work well if the waste products of cellular metabolism are not removed efficiently.

Many vitamins, minerals, and other elements of food are known to have antioxidant qualities. Some examples are: vitamins A, C, E, some B vitamins, beta-carotene, zinc, selenium, and plant compounds like lycopene, lutein, zeaxanthin, and genistein. In the sections below, the critical nutrients known to be especially important for prostate health are discussed. Most of them are antioxidants.

Essential Fatty Acids

Earlier, we briefly discussed the essential fatty acids (EFAs), omega-3 and omega-6. They are so named because the human body does not manufacture them and thus it is essential that they come from the diet. While there are many EFAs, omega-3 and omega-6 are, by far, the most critical and typically the ones subject to serious imbalances.

The human body has not changed much from prehistoric to modern man. It works best on a diet that has about a 1:1 ratio of omega-3 to omega-6. Unfortunately, unlike our prehistoric diet, modern foods—especially the highly processed ones—tend to skew this ratio. As a result, most Westerners get far too much omega-6, and far too little omega-3 in their diets.[2] This constant imbalance results in many problems including setting the stage for chronic disease processes.

In addition to the meat consumption problems described in Chapter Four, there are many other dietary items that cause the ratio of omega-6 to omega-3 to become skewed. Vegetable oils produced from corn, soy, safflower, and sunflower—the predominant oils in use today—are composed mostly of omega-6. The problem is compounded considerably when these oils are heated. High temperatures (above 300-350 degrees F.) tend to destroy the antioxidants originally present and cause oxidation and other damage to the oil, making it an additional source of unnecessary free radicals. The consequences of low omega-3 levels (or a high omega-6 to omega-3 ratio) are hormonal imbalances as well as a host of serious chronic illnesses. Studies conducted at the San Francisco VA Medical Center found that omega-6 fatty acids, such as those found in corn and similar oils, increased the growth rate of prostate cancer cells in the laboratory.[3, 4] According to the study's author, a diet high in omega-6 and low in omega-3 can turn on a cascade of events that can lead to an increased risk of developing prostate, colorectal, and some breast cancers. Another recent study by different authors confirmed a similar relationship.[5]

Some good plant sources of omega-3 are: (in order of highest omega-3 content): flaxseed, extra virgin olive oil, coconut oil, and avocados. Organic butter or cheese made from the milk of grass-fed cows is also a good source. The best animal sources are cold-water fish like salmon. Several studies have found a solid correlation between the consumption of fish oils and a decreased risk of developing prostate cancer.[6, 7, 8] Fish oil's main components are eicosapentaenoic acid (EPA), and docosahexaenoic acid (DHA), both of which are omega-3 fatty acids. One of the studies measured the blood levels of EPA and DHA from 317 men with prostate cancer, compared to 480 age-matched healthy men as controls. The men with highest levels of both had a significantly lower risk for prostate cancer as the men with the lowest levels.[9]

Omega-3 fatty acids are also abundant in most nuts and seeds, and in dark green leafy vegetables. Many of the food and herbal items that help with chronic diseases have high levels of omega-3. Omega-6 deficiencies are rare. With few exceptions, one should not take supplements containing omega-6 fatty acids. However, there are always exceptions to the rules. One essential omega-6 fatty acid, called gamma-linolenic acid or GLA, can inhibit a gene called Her-2 that is believed to be responsible for about one-third of all breast cancer cases.[10] GLA is a powerful natural remedy that has been used to treat skin problems and arthritic inflammation for many years. It is found in evening primrose, black currant seed, and borage oil. Thus, omega-6 fatty acids are not always detrimental. Remember, the human body works best when everything is in balance. Just like hormone ratios, it is the balance between omega-6 and omega-3 that is critical. Both are essential and necessary for life.

Critical Vitamins

Vitamin A — There have been numerous studies of vitamin A or retinal. Vitamin A is a fat-soluble vitamin that is needed for many functions in the body, including normal cell growth, cell reproduction, and visual acuity. Some studies have linked vitamin A deficiencies to the development of tumors while others have reported increased risk for prostate cancer with excessive vitamin A intake. Such contradictory results can be due to different sources of the vitamin. It appears that supplementary vitamin A in the form of beta-carotene obtained from plant sources reduced the size and amount of prostate tumors, while vitamin A from animal sources increased it.[11, 12] Also, beta-carotene from green or yellow vegetables was found to be significantly protective.

Niacin (Vitamin B$_3$) — Much has been written about using niacin to reduce blood cholesterol, and to help reduce blood pressure. Restoring normal blood circulation is vital to the health of all the body's tissue and organs. Niacin has a strong influence on blood vessels, causing them to dilate and increase blood flow. As a prescription medication, it is used to lower blood pressure and cholesterol levels. It is also available as a supplement and is part of the B vitamin group. Niacin comes in two forms, called niacin, and niacinamide. It is typically found in all multivitamin products, albeit not in the higher doses that are needed to reduce cholesterol levels.

Only the first form—niacin—is useful for cholesterol reduction.[13] For reducing cholesterol, a typical dosage range is about 300-1500 mg per day with meals. Again, this must be niacin, not niacinamide. Niacin is safe provided the recommended dosage is not exceeded. However, it can cause a harmless, but uncomfortable, skin flushing, particularly at higher doses. This effect can cause the skin, particularly on the extremities, to feel hot or flushed and become red. Again, this effect is harmless and typically resolves in less than one-half hour. To avoid skin flushing with niacin, divide it into smaller doses and take it with a meal.

Vitamin C — There is much evidence that vitamin C (ascorbic acid) has significant value for treating vascular problems. A daily intake of 500 mg of vitamin C (about five times the RDA) can improve blood vessel dilation. The ability of blood vessels to dilate is crucial to proper sexual performance. Studies show that vitamin C can lower blood pressure and help reduce problems with coronary artery disease, again at a dosage level of 500 mg per day.[14, 15, 16, 17] As mentioned in Chapter Five, erectile dysfunction is often the first symptom of a cardiovascular problem and may appear long before the latter is diagnosed. Any improvement in the ability of blood vessels to dilate or any lowering of blood pressure can be a major step toward restoring general health—as well as sexual function. This is particularly evident in those who smoke. Nicotine constricts blood vessels and produces free radicals that rapidly use up vitamin C, indicating that smokers are at increased risk for vitamin C deficiency.

In 2000 the food and nutrition board increased the RDA for vitamin C by about 15 mg to its current level of 75 to 90 mg, and also set a tolerable upper intake level for vitamin C at 2000 mg (2 grams). For years, natural health professionals have used doses much higher than the RDA to help resolve various conditions. The studies above and many others have shown substantial benefits to having vitamin C levels considerably higher than the RDA. In my opinion, all adults should have a daily intake of 1000-2000 mg of vitamin C from food, supplements, or both. Adequate vitamin C is particularly critical if you smoke.

Vitamin E — This vitamin is a well-known antioxidant and has been promoted as a preventive agent for several problems. It has been the subject of many studies for the prevention and amelioration of prostate disorders, and in combination with selenium (discussed later in this chapter), is probably the most valuable vitamin for prostate health.

Vitamin E comes in natural (d-alpha-tocopherol) and synthetic (dl-alpha-tocopherol) forms. The natural form is more active and is preferred. Actually, vitamin E is a family of eight slightly different molecules that are divided into two groups, tocopherols and tocotrienols. Each group contains four forms of vitamin E named alpha, beta, gamma, and delta. Many studies conclude that the d-alpha-tocopherol form of vitamin E has some ability to inhibit prostate cancer growth. Other fractions of vitamin E are not as well studied as the d-alpha-tocopherol form, but recent studies indicate they are even more powerful. A significant decrease in risk of prostate cancer is associated with the d-gamma-tocopherol form of vitamin E.[18, 19]

A study in Finland, designed to evaluate the use of vitamin E and beta-carotene for lung cancer prevention among male smokers had the unexpected result of a strong protective effect of vitamin E on the incidence of prostate cancer and mortality.[20, 21] Other studies followed the Finland study in an attempt to confirm this benefit. One concluded that while supplemental vitamin E did not appear to be associated with the risk of prostate cancer, it did appear to reduce the risk of fatal prostate cancer among current smokers and recent quitters. As I noted above, smoking depletes vitamin C. A recent study also noted a similar depletion of vitamin E that can be prevented with higher intake of Vitamin C.[22] This strongly suggests a synergistic effect between these vitamins.

Considerable evidence also exists for a synergistic relationship between vitamin E and selenium. Studies show conclusively that vitamin E and selenium are protective against both prostate and breast disorders. This synergistic relationship is particularly strong in regard to switching on the full effects of the body's apoptosis (natural cell death) machinery against cancerous growths.[23] A recent study of men with prostate cancer noted significant deficiencies of the vitamins A, C, and E, and the minerals selenium and zinc in the cancer patients as compared with healthy men.[24] Vitamin E, in particular, generally inhibits cell proliferation and enhances apoptosis in both breast and prostate cancer cells. This alteration of growth and natural cell death of dividing cells by vitamin E and selenium is significantly more effective in breast and prostate cancer than other cancers.[25, 26]

Vitamin E is actually a family of related compounds, four tocopherols and four tocotrienols. Recent research on the effects of the tocotrienol fractions strongly indicates they can help with many other problems. One study found that tocotrienols could help clear blockages in the carotid arteries (the main suppliers of blood to the brain), potentially reducing the risk of stroke.[27] Others have shown that tocotrienols can reduce the level of low-density lipoproteins (LDL), the bad form of cholesterol in the blood, as well as improve nervous system communication.[28, 29] As I mentioned in Chapter Five, narrowing of arteries in the human body do not occur in isolation. If there are deposits in the carotid arteries, then it is likely that similar problems exist in penile arteries. Thus, tocotrienols may help with erectile dysfunction caused by impaired blood circulation and clogged arteries.

The different fractions of vitamin E appear to work together (synergistically) to provide maximum benefit. Most vitamin E supplements contain only alpha-tocopherol, and this is the type of vitamin E used in most studies. In the recent past, there has been conflicting news about vitamin E in the media. Several studies found supplementation with vitamin E to be ineffective in reducing deaths from cardiovascular disease and concluded that large doses may be harmful. However, foods known to be high in natural vitamin E are protective against many diseases. One study found a protective effect against Alzheimer's disease using full spectrum vitamin E from food instead of a single fraction alpha-tocopherol supplement.[30] Studies have shown that certain foods, like nuts and certain oils, which contain copious amounts of all eight fractions of vitamin E, are highly protective against cancer. Thus, foods provide a much broader spectrum of the vitamin E components then do most over-the-counter vitamin E supplements. Excepting the past decade or so, studies of vitamin E centered on the alpha-tocopherol fraction. This likely accounts for some of the conflicting results. Unfortunately, the tocotrienol fractions of vitamin E have not been studied as extensively as the tocopherol group. However, recent research indicates tocotrienol has significant activity for the prevention of prostate and breast cancer.[31, 32, 33, 34] One study concludes:

The physiological activities of tocotrienol suggest it to be superior than alpha-tocopherol in many situations. Hence, the role of tocotrienol in the prevention of cardiovascular disease and cancer may have significant clinical implications. Additional studies on its mechanism of action, as well as, long-term intervention studies, are needed to clarify its function. From the pharmacological point-of-view, the current formulation of vitamin E supplements, which is comprised mainly of alpha-tocopherol, may be questionable.[35]

The tocopherol fractions of vitamin E may also inhibit cancer cell growth. Both alpha-tocopherol and gamma-tocopherol have been proven to be effective in controlling the growth of prostate cancer. However, gamma-tocopherol appears to offer benefits that are more significant.[36, 37] A study that compared the effects of synthetic alpha-tocopherol to natural gamma-tocopherol found that the latter inhibited prostate cancer growth at concentrations 1,000 times lower.[38]

It is important to take only natural vitamin E supplements, prefixed with "d" instead of "dl." Most over-the-counter vitamin E products, especially inexpensive ones, contain only synthetic alpha-tocopherol (dl-alpha-tocopherol). The benefits derived from taking them are, at best, marginal. Acceptable vitamin E supplements contain at least the four tocopherol components of natural vitamin E. Better supplements also have all four tocotrienol fractions derived from palm oil. Unfortunately, the latter are expensive, but then, so is treating prostate cancer! Palm oil is exceptionally high in tocotrienols and is the preferred source. It is also an excellent general-purpose oil that is stable and provides good texture and flavor. Unfortunately, when cost issues are weighed against health issues in food processing, cost issues usually win. Vegetable oils are considerably cheaper than palm, coconut, or olive oils, and are the primary oils used by both manufacturers and consumers. A discussion of the value of various oils is beyond the scope of this book, but I have provided several good references in the bibliography.

While it is best to obtain vitamin E from food products rather than supplements, it is difficult to obtain sufficient levels solely from food. However, there are many foods that are high in vitamin E. Good dietary sources of vitamin E are virtually all nuts and seeds, particularly almonds and walnuts, and oils like palm, olive, and coconut.

The prostate cancer research institute recommends a dose of 400 IU of natural vitamin E as d-alpha-tocopherol, along with 210 mg of d-gamma-tocopherol as part of its basic preventive measures.[39] In light of the latest research, it seems prudent to take a vitamin E supplement that contains all eight of the vitamin E fractions along with the above. Again, you should use only the natural form with palm oil being the preferred source. The natural tocotrienol in palm oil has also been shown to be protective for your heart.[40]

Critical Minerals

Selenium — An important dietary trace element, selenium has been found to increase immunity in a way that is protective against both breast and prostate disease. It seems selenium offers a mediating effect by actually killing cancer cells at different stages.[41, 42] Thus, selenium appears to target both nonclinical and clinical disease.* The actual way selenium does this is unclear, but studies suggest it

---

*In this context, "clinical" means that a condition has been diagnosed and medical treatment is needed. Nonclinical indicates that there has been no positive diagnosis, but the condition may still be present with minimal symptoms.

targets multiple pathways. Selenium mediates cancer cell development by preventing the cells from developing and by causing developing cancer cells to self-destruct. Many reports have confirmed
this effect making selenium a well-studied protective element
against prostate disease.[43, 44, 45, 46, 47, 48, 49] Two reports studied the
incidence of prostate disease verses selenium levels measured from
toenail clippings.[50, 51] Both confirmed that relatively high selenium
intake (compared to the current RDA) can reduce both the incidence
and risk of prostate cancer, and especially reduces the risk of developing aggressive prostate cancer.

A recent study examined the relationship between selenium
and the alpha and gamma tocopherol fractions of vitamin E. Blood
samples from 117 men who developed prostate cancer were compared to samples from a control group of 233 men. The study found
a protective effect with the alpha-tocopherol fraction of vitamin E.
However, of greater significance was the finding that men with the
highest levels of gamma-tocopherol had a five-to-one reduction in
the risk for developing prostate cancer as compared to those with
the lowest levels. Also noted was that the statistically significant
protection offered by high levels of selenium and alpha-tocopherol
occurred only when gamma-tocopherol levels were also high.[52]
This study is quite significant because it evaluated a large group of
men over a seven-year period. Synergy between various vitamin E
fractions and selenium has been noted in other studies as well.

The recommended daily intake of selenium is 55 mcg, with
an upper safe limit of 400 mcg. Many experts recommend between
100 and 200 micrograms (mcg) per day though the significant protective effect appears to be at the higher intake level. Most of the
studies I have reviewed used a level of 200 mcg. While more
research is needed to determine the optimal dose, 200 to 400 mcg
per day appears safe and prudent, particularly if little selenium is
obtained from the diet. Most seeds and nuts, as well as poultry and
eggs are high in selenium.

Zinc — is an essential trace element that plays an important
role in many body processes. Studies have found that men with
prostate disease have lower levels of zinc in their bodies than

healthy men. According to Michael Murray, N.D., the author of *Male Sexual Vitality—Chronic prostate infections are often linked to a lack of dietary zinc.* Prostate glands containing cancer generally have lower levels of zinc than healthy glands.

There are many processes in the body involved in the repair of DNA that require zinc to function properly. Since the prostate has the highest concentration of zinc of any organ in the body, it is reasonable to assume that a zinc deficiency would affect it significantly. A unique metabolic capability gives the prostate the ability to accumulate zinc. This is partially mediated by the action of the hormone, testosterone. One effect of this zinc accumulation is to inhibit abnormal growth of the prostate, primarily by increasing the rate of normal programmed cell death (apoptosis).[53] One study found a dose-response effect where supplemental zinc reduced the risk of prostate problems significantly. This same study also found a lesser, but also significant dose-response protective effect for vitamins C and E, and multi-mineral supplements.[54]

Zinc is an important regulator of many metabolic processes in the body, particularly in the prostate. One of these processes is citrate metabolism. The prostate gland accumulates and secretes extraordinarily high levels of citrate. This process is dependent on an ample supply of zinc in the prostate. In an unhealthy prostate, the ability to accumulate both zinc and citrates is altered. With BPH, zinc accumulation may be normal but citrate production may be increased. But with prostate cancer, the ability to accumulate zinc and produce citrates is impaired. As we have seen, the human body is all about balance. Studies have found that low testosterone levels generally accompany low levels of zinc and citrates in the prostate.[55, 56] Reduced zinc and poor citrate metabolism in prostatic cells, along with low testosterone levels, is characteristic of most prostate cancer.

Most foods contain small amounts of zinc. Processed foods lose most of their zinc in the processing. Legumes, seeds, and nuts contain relatively high amounts of zinc and are worthwhile additions to your diet. Pumpkin seeds in particular (see "Super Foods for the Prostate" in this chapter) are a good source of zinc. Some breakfast cereals also have reasonable amounts of zinc. The daily recommended dietary allowance (RDA) of zinc for men is 12 to 15 milligrams. But many experts recommend higher levels in the order of 25 to 80 mg/day for optimum health. As with most nutrients, older adults need more zinc than younger ones.[57] While it is best to get adequate amounts of zinc from food, this is not always possible. There has been some controversy about whether high levels of zinc supplementation (greater than 100 mg/day) negate zinc's protective effects and instead tend to impair the immune system and increase the risk of developing prostate cancer.[58, 59, 60]

Zinc and cadmium tend to occur together naturally, and some zinc supplements are not purified sufficiently to remove all traces of cadmium.[61] Cadmium is a toxic element and a known risk factor for prostate problems, and the results of some studies may have been influenced by the presence of cadmium. You should make sure zinc supplements come from reputable sources.* According to one study, zinc gluconate supplements consistently had the lowest levels of cadmium. As with most items, it is nearly impossible to overdose on nutrients from natural foods. Zinc from food sources has not been associated with an increased risk of prostate problems. Aim to get most of your zinc from food, and take only enough supplemental zinc to bring yourself to the optimal daily amount (ODA). Unfortunately, there is considerable disagreement over what the ODA for zinc should be. Until this is defined better, it is prudent to keep your total daily intake of zinc to around 50 mg per day.

Other Important Nutrients

Lycopene — Another nutrient, found in cooked tomatoes and other highly colored vegetables and berries, is lycopene. Some studies have found this nutrient to be ineffective and others have found the opposite. Probably the best answer to these conflicting results is that

---

* I have listed some websites in the appendix that perform testing on supplements for content and purity.

TABLE 1 — Approximate Lycopene Content of Various Foods*

Food	Lycopene Content (mg/100g)
Apricot, dried	0.86
Grapefruit, pink	3.36
Guava, fresh	5.40
Guava juice	3.34
Papaya, fresh	2.00–5.30
Tomatoes, fresh	0.88–4.20
Tomatoes, cooked	3.70
Tomato sauce	6.20
Tomato paste	5.40–150.00
Tomato soup, condensed	7.99
Tomato powder, dried	112.63–126.49
Tomato juice	5.00–11.60
Sun-dried tomato in oil	46.50
Watermelon, fresh	2.30–7.20

* Source: Clinton, S .K., "Lycopene: Chemistry, Biology, and Implications for Human Health and Disease," *Nutrition Review,* Vol. 56, No. 2 (Feb. 1998); 35-51.

lycopene acts synergistically with other nutrients—specifically vitamin E. A recent study found that the effects of lycopene on prostate cancer cell lines were ineffective when lycopene alone was used, but the simultaneous use of lycopene together with alpha-tocopherol (a component of vitamin E) resulted in a strong inhibitory effect against prostate cancer cell proliferation.[62] This synergistic effect was noted with some fractions of vitamin E, but not others—a strong reason for getting your vitamin E from a source that includes mixed tocopherols and tocotrienols.

It is well-known that there is a lower incidence of prostate problems in men who have a high intake of lycopene-rich foods. It appears that lycopene is best obtained from natural foods, however, and works best in the presence of other nutrients, particularly vitamin E. Lycopene is found principally in cooked tomatoes, raw strawberries, watermelon, and other brightly colored vegetables and berries, particularly those with red coloration. It has a protective benefit on prostate disease when consumed regularly from food products, but not necessarily from supplements. In one study, men who had ten or more servings of cooked tomato products had a 41 percent decrease in prostate cancer. Lower intake increased the risk proportionately.[63]

Lycopene has potent anticancer and antioxidant properties, and studies investigating it have shown a clear reduction in risk of prostate cancer development in men with high lycopene levels. Men with low lycopene levels also seem to have a higher risk of developing more aggressive cancer. Researchers at Harvard University's Medical School looked at a group of more than 47,000 male health professionals between the ages of forty and seventy-five from 1986 to 1994. The men in this group with the highest levels of lycopene in their blood were 16 percent less likely to be diagnosed with prostate cancer then the men with the lowest levels. Additionally, those with the highest levels of lycopene who did develop prostate cancer were 35 percent less likely to have aggressive cancer. Men with the higher lycopene levels also had lower PSA levels.[64, 65]

These studies and many others provide considerable evidence that high consumption of lycopene-rich natural foods can reduce the occurrence and progression of prostate disease.[66, 67, 68, 69, 70, 71] Table One shows the approximate lycopene content of various foods. Typically, foods with bright red coloration have high levels of lycopene and other potent antioxidants.

Super Foods for the Prostate

Pumpkin Seeds — For many years, the seeds of the common pumpkin have been a valuable food item in many cultures. Pumpkin seeds truly are a "super-food" for the prostate. They contain high amounts of omega-3 EFAs, protein, amino acids, iron, phosphorous, and zinc, all of which have significant value for prostate health. Historically, pumpkin seeds have been used in many cultures, including Native Americans, to eliminate intestinal parasites and to treat BPH and prostatitis. There is evidence that they may also help control prostate cancer. Unfortunately, while there is extensive anecdotal and historical evidence regarding the use of pumpkin seeds for prostate problems, I could only find one specific related clinical study. Fifty-three men with BPH participated in this double-blind study, and it concluded that urinary flow, residual urine, urgency and frequency of urination—all symptoms of BPH—were significantly improved in the treatment group.[72]

Historical evidence of the beneficial effects of pumpkin seeds is strong enough that many European countries have formally approved them for treatment of BPH. Germany's commission E has also approved them for other urinary problems. Pumpkin seeds have extremely high zinc content.

For years, our fat-conscious society has scared many of us away from seeds and nuts since most have relatively high fat content. As we have seen, however, not all fats are created equal. Seeds and nuts are likely the most nutritious foods on the planet. They are nutrient-dense foods. Although most have high fat content, their fat consists almost exclusively of the healthy variety. One of the causes of chronic illness in our western society is that people eat too few foods with high nutrient content, opting instead for nutrient-poor foods and snacks. For example, one ounce of pumpkin seeds contains about 150 calories and nearly 10 grams of protein. A typical one-ounce chocolate chip cookie has about the same number of calories, but less than two grams of protein and little in the way of other nutrients. Table 2 shows a comparison of some critical minerals in each, making it easy to see which is the better snack.

In addition to higher protein and mineral levels, pumpkin seeds contain no cholesterol and no hydrogenated or artificial fats. They are high in protective compounds called phytosterols and other chemicals known as cucurbitacins that tend to inhibit some of the transformation of testosterone to dihydrotestosterone (DHT). As we learned in Chapter Four, excess DHT is associated with prostate

TABLE 2 — Comparison of the mineral content (in mg) of
Pumpkin Seeds and a Cookie*

Mineral Name	Pumpkin Seeds	Chocolate Chip Cookie
Calcium	12	2
Iron	4.25	.72
Magnesium	152	10
Phosphorus	333	16
Potassium	229	28
Zinc	2.12	.14
Copper	.39	.04

*Source: Corinne T. Netzer, The Complete Book of Vitamin and Mineral Counts
(Dell Publishing, 1997)

dysfunction, particularly BPH and possibly cancer. Pumpkin seeds
are also a good source of L-tryptophan, an amino acid in which many
people are deficient and can help with sleep problems and depression.
It is best to purchase raw, organic seeds, preferably unsalted.

Other Nuts and Seeds — All nuts and seeds are nutritionally rich foods with high levels of beneficial fats, minerals, vitamins, and plant sterols. Walnuts and peanuts in particular improve
overall circulation and thus are beneficial for the prostate. Both help
to reverse a problem called endothelial dysfunction. Endothelial tissue is a thin flat layer of cells that lines virtually all blood vessels in
the body. Dysfunction in this tissue is directly associated with atherosclerosis, cardiovascular disease, and erectile dysfunction, as
well as many other circulatory problems. Peanuts also help reduce
dysfunction in this tissue due to their high amino acid content, particularly L-arginine. While most other nuts and seeds are beneficial,
walnuts and peanuts are particularly effective.[73, 74, 75] The relationship of endothelial dysfunction to erectile dysfunction is discussed
in more detail in Chapter Nine.

Cruciferous vegetables — In recent years there has been much media attention about the cruciferous vegetable family (broccoli, cauliflower, brussels sprouts, cabbage, and watercress) regarding their ability to offer protection against various cancers. There is little question that a diet high in vegetables is health-inducing and protective against all types of cancer. Hundreds of clinical studies over many years have confirmed this conclusively. Vegetables in the cruciferous family—like most other vegetables—are high in nutrients. There are special chemicals in the cruciferous family, particularly in broccoli, which may help eliminate carcinogens before they do damage.* Solid evidence indicates that cruciferous vegetables inhibit certain cancers, like lung and colorectal cancer, but the evidence for prostate (and breast) cancer is not as conclusive. Studies have demonstrated that chemicals in this vegetable family can induce cell death in prostate cancer cell lines in the laboratory.[76, 77, 78, 79, 80] Other studies found that men with prostate cancer reported a significantly lower intake of cruciferous vegetables then men who were cancer free.[81, 82, 83, 84] In one study, men who consumed more than three servings of cruciferous vegetables per week had a 41 percent lower risk of developing prostate cancer than men who consumed less than one serving per week.[85] Conversely, some studies found no statistically significant protective effect against prostate cancer for the cruciferous vegetable family.[86, 87]

What is the net result of all this? Remember, clinical studies are looking for provable, statistically significant results. As I mentioned earlier, it is often quite difficult to determine a connective relationship between a disease and a food item with absolute certainty. There is solid evidence that vegetables in the cruciferous family have a significant protective effect for some cancers. And there is also considerable suggestive evidence that a similar effect occurs with prostate and breast cancer. A recent meta-analysis of the studies above and others came to the conclusion that there is evidence that vegetables in the cruciferous family are protective

---

*Carcinogens are defined as chemicals known to cause cancer.

against prostate cancer.*[88] It is not the concrete, obvious, or conclusive evidence we would like, but it is there. The bottom line is that the data is in favor of a protective role for vegetables in this family. So, eat your broccoli—at least a few servings per week!

Green Tea, White Tea, and Black Tea — The power of all tea varieties comes from their ample allotment of substances called polyphenols or catechins. These are antioxidant plant chemicals that tend to neutralize the damaging effects of free radicals. Green Tea contains a polyphenol called Epigallocatechin gallate (EGCG) that has been shown to benefit certain blood cancers, like leukemia. Black and white teas also have an abundance of potent antioxidants that help lower oxidation of LDL-cholesterol, resulting in a decreased risk of such deposits blocking blood flow. In one study healthy men who drank tea had measurable increases in cardiac blood flow after consumption. There was little difference noted in the different types of teas.[89] As discussed in Chapter Five, anything that aids in decreasing the amount of arterial plaque deposits can increase blood circulation, and any such increase can help reduce problems with erectile dysfunction.[90, 91]

Free radicals can damage the DNA that allows cells to reproduce. This is believed to cause cell mutations that lead to the runaway growth of cancer. Tea also helps diminish formation of free radicals resulting in a decreased risk of some specific cancers, including prostate cancer. In a recent Chinese study it was noted that drinking three or more cups of green tea daily had a significant protective effect against prostate cancer. The men who drank the most tea, for the longest time, had the highest level of protection.[92] Tea helps protect the prostate from developing cancer and can also help reduce existing tumor size by increasing destruction of cancerous cells. This is not to say that drinking tea will cure prostate or other cancers, but there is substantial evidence that the polyphenols in tea are protective against cancerous growths.[93, 94, 95]

At the annual meeting of the American Association for Cancer Research, in Anaheim, California, in April 2005, Dr. Saverio

---

* A meta-analysis is a statistical analysis of many separate but related studies.

Bettuzzi, associate professor of biochemistry at the School of Medicine, University of Parma, Italy, presented the results of his recent study. He studied sixty-two men who were already at high risk of developing prostate cancer due to precancerous prostate lesions. Such lesions often develop into prostate cancer within a year. Thirty-two of the men were given a pill containing 200 mg of green tea cachechins to take three times a day for a year. The other thirty men (controls) were given a placebo. At the end of the study, only one man in the green tea group developed prostate cancer. In the control group, nine men developed cancer.[96]

It is well-known that Japanese men have a low rate of prostate cancer. While there are many differences in culture and diet between Japanese and American men, one significant difference is the amount of plant sterols consumed from tea and other sources. The Japanese consume many times what Americans do. It appears prudent to add a cup or two of green, black, or white tea to your daily routine.

Soy Products — In the recent past there has been a wealth of positive information in the media about soy. The triggering factor for this news is that numerous studies have found lower rates of prostate and breast cancer in Asian countries, where soy is consumed liberally. Products made from soy have enjoyed a reputation for their genistein isoflavone compounds that have been shown to be mildly effective in promoting cancer cell death in the laboratory. Much of this can likely be attributed to the fact that soy products contain high levels of vitamin E, particularly the gamma-tocopherol fraction, which (as discussed earlier in this chapter), is protective against prostate cancer. However, while there are many soy products on the market, there is little independent science that shows any major benefit. Also, most of the soy products available in the United States are highly processed with large amounts of sugar and other ingredients that have a negative effect on health. Unfortunately, the overall impact is that much of the positive news on soy is more advertising hype than science. Some research also suggests that soy products can depress thyroid function. Depressed thyroid function (hypothyroidism) is often associated with prostate and erectile dysfunction. It is possible that this relates to an imbalance in the sex steroid hormones caused by the hypothyroidism. In a recent advisory, the American Heart Association concluded that,

> The efficacy and safety of soy isoflavones for preventing or treating cancer of the breast, endometrium, and prostate are not established; evidence from clinical trials is meager and cautionary with regard to a possible adverse effect. For this reason, use of isoflavone supplements in food or pills is not recommended. Thus, earlier research indicating that soy protein has clinically important favorable effects as compared with other proteins has not been confirmed.[97]

While natural soy products in the diet like tofu may be helpful, it is not prudent to take soy extracts in the hope of helping resolve prostate conditions. It is always best to steer clear of highly processed soy products.

Flaxseed — The isoflavones in flaxseed seem to have potent preventive roles in the treatment of breast and prostate cancers.[98] Recently, considerable attention has been devoted to flax oil and seed. Generally, any food rich in isoflavones has properties that can help prevent cancer cells from multiplying.

Flaxseed is also high in phytoestrogens. As described earlier, phytoestrogens have chemical structures and properties similar to that of human estrogens. To a weak extent they can mimic or modulate estrogen metabolism. They exert hormonal effects similar to human estrogens, but without the negative potential of excess estrogen exposure. Soy and flaxseed have both been shown to be abundant in such phytoestrogens. There is an inherent structural similarity between the phytoestrogens genistein and daidzein that are found in soy, and the phytoestrogens enterolactone and enterodiol in flaxseed. However, supplementation with flaxseed has a greater estrogen modulation effect than soy. This is important since estrogen modulation via phytoestrogens has a profound effect on prostate and breast disorders, including cancer.[99] Interestingly, this shift in estrogen metabolism towards the phytoestrogens—which are less biologically active—does not have a negative effect on bone cell metabolism, leading to the conclusion that blocking estrogens produced by the body with phytoestrogens does not increase the risk of developing osteoporosis.

Another major advantage of using flax supplements over soy is a reduction in the level of prostate specific antigen (PSA), which is produced only by the prostate and is generally accepted to be an indicator of disease (particularly cancer) progression. PSA levels tend to be elevated in cancerous prostates, but can also be elevated by prostatitis or BPH, albeit usually not to the same high levels as with prostate cancer. In one study, 25 men scheduled for surgery to have cancerous prostates removed consumed 30 grams/day (about 3 heaping tablespoons) of flaxseed and restricted their fat intake until the date of surgery.[100] Aside from a lowering of PSA levels, it was also noted that tumor cells did not divide as quickly in the men on the diet and there was a greater rate of tumor cell apoptosis in this group. It was also noted that cholesterol levels dropped during the study period. However, the researchers added that this effect might also be due to the low-fat diet.

Flaxseed is also high in omega-3 fatty acids and it can provide benefit by balancing other higher order fats, particularly omega-6. The fiber and omega-3 fatty acids contained in flax can also lower blood pressure and reduce risks of coronary events. Flaxseed can be purchased in most health food stores and some grocery stores. Most stores also sell flax oil but it is better to consume flax from freshly ground seed rather than oil. Flax oil has a tendency to become rancid; a long transition time from extraction of the oil to consumption may render the oil more harmful than beneficial. One study found that flax oil might actually increase prostate problems. Flax oil is high in Alpha-linolenic acid (ALA)—an essential nutrient associated with cardiovascular benefits, but the study concluded that while a high intake of ALA did not appear to increase overall risk of developing prostate cancer, it did increase the risk of developing *aggressive* prostate cancer.[101] Raw flaxseed has a lower ALA content than flax oil and several studies have shown it to be protective against prostate cancer. Raw, unbroken flaxseed will store almost indefinitely without becoming rancid and does not need refrigeration. A good way to use it is to sprinkle a tablespoon or two of ground flaxseed on some salad or cereal.

Summary

I have presented considerable information about various nutrients and foods, items that form a basic nutrient group that all men should include in their diets. Reference books, such as those by Corinne Netzer (see bibliography) can give you information about the nutrient content of the foods you eat. Use them and the guidelines in this chapter to determine how much of each nutrient you are getting. If the amount from your food is less than the recommended level, make up the balance with supplements. The foods and supplements are helpful regardless of the health of your prostate and can help to reverse existing prostate problems. If you are lucky enough to have a healthy prostate, they can help you keep it that way. There are many other items that can also help alleviate prostate problems. In the next chapter, we will discuss the action of various herbs for that purpose.

Chapter Eight

Herbal Help for Prostate Dysfunction

The use of medicinal plants has a history that stretches back several thousand years. In many areas of the world, herbal medicine is the primary—and often the only—treatment for many health conditions. It is interesting to note that approximately 95 percent of pharmaceuticals used in the United States and Western Europe are derived from plants. For the purpose of securing a patent, pharmaceutical manufacturers use plant chemicals as templates to create synthetic substitutes. Unfortunately, such substances rarely have exactly the same characteristics as nature's original, and often they cause unrelated side effects.

Sadly, our wide range of powerful pharmaceuticals has not elevated our overall health, particularly with regard to chronic illnesses. On the contrary, to many observers it appears instead to have hastened our decline. Comparing overall health, the United States ranks just barely above a "D" grade compared to other civilized countries, particularly in handling of chronic illnesses like prostate dysfunction. Medications for chronic conditions often have significant undesirable side effects frequently causing patients to stop using them. Herbal medications typically have less undesirable side effects, and in many cases support body functions in a way that improves overall health. This chapter concentrates on herbs that have known medicinal value for prostate problems. Most have few, if any, side effects.

Many herbs have both nutritional and medicinal properties, and their effects span a range from mild to quite strong. Often, there is little difference between a medicinal herb and a food, and the separation is arbitrary. Many can be either, and they are differentiated only by their traditional use. For example, in the previous chapter pumpkin seeds were treated as a food. This definition holds when you eat them casually. However, when using them to alleviate prostate dysfunction, they could be considered to be medicinal. Garlic, for example, is obviously a popular food item and it is also a medicinal herb. If you use it for its taste, it is called a food. But if you use it to help lower your blood pressure or cholesterol levels, you are using it as a medicinal herb. The same is true of many herbs.

Some herbs are used only medicinally, and rarely, or never, eaten as food. Obviously, with herbs commonly used as food items—like pumpkin seeds and garlic—you can usually consume as much as you like without risk of ill effects or overdose. However, herbs used strictly for their medicinal effects can be dangerous if misused. In the chapters that follow, there are warnings where excessive use of an item can have adverse effects.

Phytochemicals

All plants contain thousands of nutrients in the form of vitamins, minerals, and other chemicals. Collectively, these plant constituents are called *phytochemicals*. "Phyto" is a Greek work meaning "plant." All plants naturally produce phytochemicals. They function as agents that protect the plant from fungi, disease, and insects. Many of them are antioxidants. When consumed by humans, they enhance the body's natural defenses and are health promoting and protective against chronic illness. There are many groups of phytochemicals—far more than we can discuss here. Regarding prostate health, we are concerned primarily with the subgroups of phytochemicals known as phytoestrogens and phytosterols.

Phytoestrogens are plant-based chemicals that mimic the action of human estrogens in many ways. Human estrogens—specifically estrone and estradiol—can follow a metabolic pathway that leads to promoting excessive cell growth, which may result in BPH or cancer. Phytoestrogens do not undergo such a transformation. They are found in various quantities in virtually all plants and abundant in most seeds, nuts, fruits, berries, and vegetables. As we discussed in Chapter Three, the prostate contains receptors for several hormones. These receptors respond to stimulation by estrogen, progesterone, testosterone, DHT, and other hormones. Phytoestrogens attach to estrogen receptors on the prostate and by doing so, block some of the negative effects of estrogen on prostate growth. A high intake of plant-based phytoestrogens can reduce the risk of prostate problems.[1]

Phytoestrogens consist mainly of substances called lignans and isoflavonoids. Lignans are found in whole-grain bread, seeds, berries, and vegetables, and isoflavonoids are found in flaxseed, soy, many teas, and many herbs. Another class of phytoestrogens is coumestans, which are found primarily in cruciferous vegetables like broccoli. In Japan, which has a very low rate of prostate and breast cancer, the consumption of phytoestrogens from soy, tea, and other plant products is quite high.

A recent study reviewed the incidence of prostate cancer in Finland, the United States, and Japan, with respect to intake of phytoestrogens.[2] The Finns had a lower incidence of prostate cancer than the U.S., which is interesting considering their typical high-fat dietary intake. However, the Finns typically have high dietary intake of lignans and isoflavonoids from whole-grain bread, berries, seeds, and vegetables that appear to help override the risks of their high-fat diet. The incidence of prostate cancer in both the United States and Finland is considerably higher than that in Japan. In this study, the Japanese subjects ate a traditional diet and had significantly higher levels of isoflavonoids in their urine than did the other subjects. The study concluded that dietary phytoestrogens have a strong role as protective compounds with regard to prostate disease.

Phytosterols are plant fats that are essentially in the same family as steroids.* Chemically similar to cholesterol, they are

---

* Phytosterols are also known as sterols and sterolins.

found in all plant-based foods. They have immune-enhancing effects on the body as well as a profound effect on the prostate without the negative effects of steroids. The highest concentrations of phytosterols are found in plant oils, seeds and nuts, and certain berries.[3]

The most well-studied phytosterol is beta-sitosterol. It is the major phytosterol in many herbs and foods with proven value for prostate dysfunction. Beta-sitosterol is quite similar (chemically) to cholesterol but is absorbed at a much lower rate by the body. Studies have shown that an intake of 130-160 mg per day can lower cholesterol levels in humans.[4, 5, 6] This is likely part of the reason beta-sitosterol is health inducing. Many of the herbs discussed in this chapter and the next are known to have high levels of beta-sitosterol, and many of the referenced studies have used beta-sitosterol extracts separately or as part of herbal combinations.

A Note on Synergy

Professional herbalists often treat prostate and erectile dysfunction with several herbs simultaneously. They know that the chemical constituents of many herbs—and foods—act synergistically and often have significantly greater benefit when used together. For prostate problems, beta-sitosterol is one of the potent components of herbs known to help. In my opinion, extracting and concentrating it from herbal sources is not always advantageous. In nature, nutrients are never found in isolation. Purifying one component of an herb for medicinal purposes is akin to producing a pharmaceutical drug and sometimes results in unintended consequences. For example, the bark of the white willow tree contains a chemical called salicin, which the body converts to salicylic acid. Extracts of salicylic acid from white willow bark were originally used to make aspirin (acetylsalicylic acid). Willow bark and aspirin are similar in their pain-relieving properties. However, gastrointestinal problems are virtually nonexistent with willow bark, but are a serious problem with aspirin. Other components in willow bark seem to work synergistically to mediate its effects on the stomach and intestinal tract, thus preventing negative side effects.

Synergy between herbs is extremely important and is typically what makes herbal combinations much more powerful. All herbalists know this. I believe that using the synergy of herbal combinations is a much better way of achieving a successful outcome than extracting specific components of individual herbs. While I discuss each herb separately, keep in mind that many of the herbs have broad beneficial effects that overlap.

Saw Palmetto (Serenoa repens)

Traditionally, saw palmetto has been the choice of natural practitioners for treatment for BPH. It is a well-studied herb that has proven value for BPH and may possibly help reduce tumor size in prostate cancer. It has also shown value in treating erectile dysfunction. Saw palmetto is a bush-like, dwarf palm that grows mostly in the southern United States. The medicinal part of the plant is its small bluish-purple berries. They have a long history of use for prostate problems, particularly BPH, and are quite safe.

As we have shown, 5-alpha-reductase is the enzyme that converts testosterone to DHT, and DHT is partially responsible for initiating growth of the prostate. Inhibiting this enzyme also appears to have a positive effect on wound healing, especially in older men.[7] While the exact mechanism of saw palmetto is not known, it is believed it inhibits the 5-alpha-reductase enzyme. A commercial product called Permixon—an extract of saw palmetto—is widely used in Europe for treating BPH. Studies of Permixon (and similar products) have shown significant improvement in maximum urinary flow, a decrease in overall prostate size, and improvement in other symptoms including sexual function. However, while symptom improvements were noted at six months, the maximum benefits of treatment were not evident until the second year.[8, 9] One study noted that sexual function remained stable during the first year of treatment but improved significantly during the second year.[10] This suggests that treatment with saw palmetto may initiate a long-term healing process within the prostate.[11]

Saw palmetto has been well-studied both in the United States and in other countries. A meta-analysis published in the *Journal of the American Medical Association* in 1998 evaluated a total of eighteen controlled studies involving 2,939 men that met the author's inclusion criteria. This analysis concluded that saw palmetto produced improvements in urinary tract symptoms and urinary flow rate without the side effects associated with the popular prescription drug, Finasteride.[12] Another, more recent meta-analysis confirmed the original results.[13]

Saw palmetto has very few side effects, and many men report that it enhances libido, although this has not been shown conclusively by any studies. It is quite possible, however, that the reduction in prostate size and the improvement of overall urinary health could result in a feeling of well being that could easily account for the increased libido.

It is important to use a standardized extract of saw palmetto berries. Some supplement manufacturers sell the ground berries of saw palmetto in capsule form. While the berries are indeed healthy, to see significant improvement in prostate problems you would need to swallow a significant number of capsules. In this case, it is more effective to use a concentrated and standardized extract. Also, virtually all studies of saw palmetto that have shown improvement in prostate symptoms have used only such extracts. When you are purchasing a saw palmetto extract, look for the words "standardized to contain 85-95 percent fatty acids and sterols" on the label. The dosage that has proven effective is 320 mg per day divided into two doses of 160 mg or four doses of 80 mg.

While saw palmetto is effective by itself, it is even more effective when used along with other herbs, like pygeum and nettle (described below), and pumpkin seeds (discussed in Chapter Seven). Many supplement manufacturers provide products combining saw palmetto extract with pygeum, pumpkin seed oil, and nettle. Synergy is one of nature's most powerful effects but it is not always easy to study, though it has gained more attention recently.

Pygeum (Pygeum africanum, Prunus africana)

Pygeum grows primarily in Africa and is commonly called the African prune tree. Its bark has traditionally been used for the treatment of urinary and prostate problems. A meta-analysis looked at eighteen randomized, controlled trials using extracts of pygeum. These trials included a total of 1,562 men with BPH.[14] The review concluded that the studies show pygeum improves the urinary symptoms of BPH with few side effects. In these studies, men using pygeum were more than twice as likely to report improvement in overall symptoms. In Europe, a pygeum africanus extract is available as a commercial product known as Tadenan. Two European studies treated a total of 348 men with this extract at a dose rate of 50 mg twice daily for two months.[15, 16] Significant improvements were noted after the two-month treatment period, particularly in nighttime voiding, a persistently annoying symptom of BPH. Nocturnal frequency was reduced by 32 percent, and urinary flow and volume were also significantly improved. One interesting observation of the first study was that the beneficial effect of Pygeum appeared to last for at least one month after the two-month trial period. Other studies have indicated that, like saw palmetto, the full effects of supplementing with pygeum are only obtained after a period of use of at least six months.

Pygeum seems to be effective at a dosage of about 100 mg per day. Adverse effects of pygeum are rare and mild. The most common side effect appears to be mild gastrointestinal disturbances that often resolve after a few weeks of continuous use. There does not appear to be any toxic effects.

Pygeum does not seem to affect the prostate with quite the same mechanism of action as saw palmetto, although it is similar. While pygeum is sometimes used alone, more often it is used in combination with saw palmetto and other herbs for the synergistic effect. Unfortunately, as with many herbs, studies are small and limited to short durations due to financial considerations, but the evidence is quite strong that pygeum significantly improves symptoms of BPH.[17, 18, 19]

Stinging Nettle Root (Urtica dioica)

Stinging nettle (or simply nettle) is a weed-like plant that grows wild throughout the United States. It has a long history of therapeutic use for many different health issues. Both the root and the leaves of the plant are used medicinally.

There are different types of nettle products, some made from the leaves of the plant and others from the root. The leaves and other above-ground parts of the nettle plant have different chemical components from those of the root, and thus different medicinal properties. Both root and leaves have anti-inflammatory properties that make them effective for reducing chronic prostatitis but nettle root appears to be more effective at treating BPH. The mechanism of action of nettle root is not completely known, but it is believed that it inhibits both the 5-alpha-reductase and aromatase enzymes. As discussed earlier, reducing 5-alpha-reductase and aromatase results in lowered levels of both DHT and estrogen, which are believed to increase risk of prostate cancer and BPH. It also appears that nettle reduces the level of sex hormone binding globulin (SHBG) causing a slight increase in free testosterone which is also beneficial.[20, 21]

Like saw palmetto and pygeum, nettle contains many phytosterols that can help relieve symptoms of prostate dysfunction. Studies have shown that nettle by itself is not quite as effective as saw palmetto or pygeum in treating BPH, though it is usually combined with both for its synergistic effect. A Japanese study concluded that the plant sterols in nettle root inhibited activity of certain prostate cells in such a way as to help prevent the excess growth of BPH.[22] A large, long-term, double-blind study in Germany also confirmed its usefulness in treating BPH.[23] In another study, extracts of nettle root were observed to have an inhibitory effect on the proliferation of human prostate cancer cells in the laboratory.[24] In animals induced in the laboratory to have a four times the normal prostate tissue, nettle reduced the excess tissue by more than one-third.[25]

Nettle has a long history of successful use. It is a highly valued medicinal plant and is used for a variety of conditions. Nettle leaf, used as a tea, has a long and well-documented historical use both as a diuretic and as an anti-inflammatory. Nettle tea is quite effective at reducing the joint pain and inflammation associated with arthritis. Its diuretic properties can also help reduce blood pressure, and as we have discussed above, nettle root is quite useful for reducing symptoms associated with BPH. The recommended dose of nettle extract is between 600 and 1200 mg per day. When made into a tea, about a tablespoon of either leaves or root can be put into a tea strainer and steeped in eight ounces of water for five to ten minutes. In some cultures, nettle leaves are cooked and eaten like spinach.

Flower Pollen Extracts

For many years, extracts of flower pollen have been used in Europe to treat BPH and prostatitis. Flower pollen is a concentrated, allergen-free extract of the male seeds of ryegrass and various other flowering plants. In Europe a commercial flower pollen extract named Cernilton is well studied. Products produced by other manufacturers are similar and are usually marketed as Swedish flower pollen or simply, flower pollen. While this supplement is widely accepted in Europe, it has just begun to make an appearance in the United States.

Flower pollen extract appears to work via multiple chemical pathways to reduce the severity of both BPH and prostatitis. Several studies have shown significant statistical improvements in urinary flow, intermittent voiding, dribbling, the number of times one wakes up at night to urinate (nocturia), and urinary retention.[26, 27, 28, 29] A reduction in symptoms can often occur relatively quickly, but as with most herbal remedies for the prostate, the full effect may not be seen immediately. In a study of seventy-nine patients, 85 percent noted improvements in symptoms within the twelve-week study interval. During this initial phase, no changes were noted in prostate size. However, when the study was extended to one year, twenty-eight patients—approximately 35 percent—showed a mean decrease in prostate volume of about 20 percent.[30] Thus, the benefits of flower pollen may be ongoing over a much longer period than typically considered, again suggesting that it may be initiating a long-term healing process. One prominent manufacturer recommends a minimum use of six months.

Chronic prostatitis is a difficult condition to treat, but it does appear to respond to treatment with flower pollen. White blood cells in the urine after a prostate massage are a good general indicator of an active prostate infection or prostatitis. One study noted a reduction in these cells after using flower pollen. This same study noted that treatment with flower pollen resulted in a favorable response in 78 percent of the patients treated, with 42 percent improving significantly, and 36 percent having near total resolution of their symptoms. The authors of the study cautioned that these favorable results occurred only on men without other prostate or urinary complications.[31]

While there is no clinical evidence of flower pollen helping to reverse prostate cancer, substances have been found in flower pollen that inhibited the growth of the prostate cells involved in BPH.[32] In addition some studies showed an inhibitory effect on the growth of prostate cancer cells in the laboratory.[33, 34]

Flower pollen, due to its significant positive effects on the prostate, is now gaining popularity in the United States. None of the studies I reviewed indicated any adverse side effects of its use. The dosage used in most of the studies is about 250 mg of standardized extract per day, divided into two doses. However, that dosage is specific to the product tested, which was, in most cases, the particular brand named Cernilton. A supplemental flower pollen extract should be standardized to contain a minimum of 1.4 percent alpha amino acids and 0.08 percent phytosterols. At that standardization, one manufacturer (Source Naturals) recommends a dosage of 378 mg per day, divided into three doses. Regardless of which brand you choose, you should see results in a few weeks. Men who are particularly sensitive to it can see results in as little as a few days, and benefits may continue to accumulate with time. Maximum benefit may not be seen for a year or more. This strongly suggests that it is slowly improving the overall health of the prostate.

Garlic

Garlic is one of several edible plants of the genus allium in the lily family. Some other edible plants in this family are chives, leeks, onions, scallions, and shallots. For thousands of years in virtually every culture, garlic and the other members of this group have been used both as food and medicine. These vegetables contain a number of substances proven to have healthful benefits for prostate problems. Several studies have shown garlic (and other vegetables in this family) to have powerful anti-tumor properties.[35, 36, 37, 38] In a recent, relatively large study of men with and without prostate cancer, men who consumed more than ten grams per day of allium vegetables had about a 50 percent lower risk of prostate cancer than those who consumed less than about two grams per day.[39]

Garlic has also been shown to reduce blood pressure and cholesterol levels and increase blood circulation in both animals and humans. These are all of critical importance in preventing diabetes, heart disease, dementia, as well as prostate problems like ED.[40, 41] One way it appears to do this is by helping to increase nitric oxide levels—a chemical that is responsible for increasing blood flow through the body. Nitric oxide is discussed in more detail in Chapters Nine and Ten.

Garlic can be consumed in many ways. You can mix it with almost any food, and it can be eaten cooked or raw. Medicinally, the best way to consume garlic is by taking one to three cloves and crushing them. (Small garlic crushers are available in many food stores.) After crushing the cloves, let them to sit for about five minutes to allow the active constituents to mix. The crushed garlic can then be combined with an ounce or two of fruit juice and swallowed. This technique lets you get a relatively high dose of garlic in your digestive system without giving you a bad case of "garlic breath." Other ways to take garlic are to purchase an aged extract as a supplement. However, in my experience the crushed raw garlic is more powerful and effective. Regardless of how you take it, adding garlic and the other allium vegetables to your diet on a regular basis can improve your health dramatically.

Ginkgo (Ginkgo Biloba)

Traditional Chinese herbalists have used Ginkgo for many years. It is also known in folklore as the maidenhair tree. Ginkgo is one of the oldest living tree species and has been used by Chinese herbalists for thousands of years. The part of the plant used is its leaves. It is well researched and has become one of the top selling medicinal herbs worldwide. Ginkgo's proven effectiveness in improving blood circulation throughout the body also makes it a useful herb for overcoming the circulation problems inherent with most prostate dysfunction. Few studies have been done on ginkgo specifically with respect to prostate disorders except some for reversing sexual dysfunction induced by antidepressants and other prescription drugs.[42, 43] These studies had conflicting results, with one showing ginkgo to be significantly effective in overcoming the dysfunction, and the other showing little positive results. However, both studies were of short duration, and the positive effects from ginkgo—like other herbal remedies discussed in this chapter—may take up to a year to become evident.

Ginkgo is known to improve blood circulation throughout the body. Additional blood flow in the area of the prostate is bound to be helpful for its general health. Extracts of ginkgo are included in many men's health supplements for its ability to promote healthy circulation, which is imperative for maintaining a healthy prostate gland. Studies have shown ginkgo to have a variety of effects on the body. This includes antioxidant action as a free radical scavenger, a relaxing effect on vascular walls, improved blood flow, and stimulation of neurotransmitters. One recent study of mice with breast or brain cancer showed a decrease in a cell receptor associated with invasive cancer after treatment with ginkgo.[44] In another, the author wrote:

> Ginkgo shows a very strong scavenging action on free radicals, and is thus considered to be useful for the treatment of diseases related to the production of free radicals, such as ischemic heart disease, cerebral infarction, chronic inflammation, and aging.[45] *

In Europe ginkgo is used for treating many different problems including impaired memory, tinnitus (ringing in the ears), and dizziness, all of which can be caused by insufficient blood flow to the brain. In addition, a significant body of research currently underway is showing promise for the possibility of long-term ginkgo use to help delay or prevent the onset of Alzheimer's disease.

Ginkgo is generally regarded as extremely safe, has few side effects, and can be taken for long periods of time.[46] One of gingko's effects is to thin the blood, so it should not be taken by anyone who is anticipating surgery in the immediate future, or is using prescription blood-thinning medication.

Gingko is a bulky herb. It takes a lot of leaf to make a useful amount. Typical gingko preparations are concentrated 50:1 extracts, meaning that it takes fifty ounces of leaf to produce one ounce of product. Use only gingko produced by a reputable manufacturer that is at least a 50:1 extract and standardized to contain at least 24 percent flavonglycosides and 6 percent terpene lactones. A typical dosage of such an extract is 120 mg per day divided into two or four doses.

---

* Ischemia is a shortage of oxygen due to insufficient blood flow. Ischemic heart disease is due to a decrease in blood supply to the heart, usually by constriction or obstruction of the arteries leading to the heart. Cerebral infarction is the medical term for a stroke.

Beta-Sitosterol

Beta-sitosterol is not an herb but a ubiquitous plant sterol. It is abundant in all the herbs discussed in this chapter and found in virtually all vegetables and plants that humans eat. Herbs like saw palmetto and pygeum as well as foods like pumpkin seeds contain high amounts of beta-sitosterol. Some books tout the benefits of beta-sitosterol and undoubtedly it is a key player in nearly all the herbs discussed in this book. As mentioned earlier, it is my belief that attempting to separate a single active ingredient from various herbs to treat prostate dysfunction is a futile process—akin to trying to produce an herbal "silver bullet." Granted, beta-sitosterol is an active component in all of these herbs, but using it alone, as some of these books recommend, is, in my opinion, ignoring the complimentary effects of other ingredients in the plant. For example, while garlic is certainly a health food, you would not want it as the only ingredient in a meal.

In one study, two hundred men with BPH were treated with the phytosterol beta-sitosterol and followed for six months using a variety of laboratory tests as well as symptom evaluations. The active treatment of 20 mg of beta-sitosterol three times daily was given to half the group while the others received a placebo. The treated group improved in both subjective symptoms of BPH and objective measurement of improved urine flow. An interesting note from this study is that a popular German herbal preparation for the treatment of BPH has been sold since about 1975 under the trade name, Harzol. It contains a mixture of phytoestrogens and phytosterols including a high quantity of beta-sitosterol. Harzol is made from saw palmetto, pygeum, and other herbs.[47] Other studies noted similar benefits for beta-sitosterol.[48, 49, 50]

Beta-sitosterol supplements are produced from various plants like soybeans and sugar cane. Typically, they contain anywhere from 100 to 400 mg of beta-sitosterol per capsule along with other phytosterols. The usual dosage of beta-sitosterol is about 300 mg per day. Such supplements can be effective for prostate dysfunction when used for a few months in the initial treatment of BPH or prostatitis. Beta-sitosterol is also effective at helping to lower cholesterol levels, and can augment the actions of the other herbs discussed above. However, for long-term use, unless you have a specific need to lower cholesterol levels, the herbs mentioned above will provide ample phytosterols, including beta-sitosterol, for prostate problems.

Modified Citrus Pectin

Modified Citrus Pectin is a commercially available supplement that shows promise in the treatment of prostate cancer. Pectin is a protein found in the first part of the plant cell wall to be formed as a plant grows and is abundant in the rinds of citrus fruit. It is generally not absorbed well into the bloodstream of humans in its raw form, but it can be more easily absorbed when structurally modified into a smaller molecule. Thus, "modified citrus pectin" is a form of pectin that has been cut and chemically reformed into smaller molecular units that the body can absorb easier.

Certain types of cancer cells, particularly those of prostate cancer, have a group of molecular receptors on their outer surfaces that enable the cancer cells to bind together and grow. Modified citrus pectin appears to be able to bind to these receptors, blocking them from initiating the action that causes the cancer to grow and spread. In a landmark animal study, citrus pectin was shown to have a significant ability to block the spread of prostate cancer.[51] In this study, rats with prostate cancer were given modified citrus pectin in their water. The treated rats had significantly less cancer metastasis to their lungs than the non-treated rats. The modified citrus pectin did not appear to have any effect on the growth of the primary prostate tumors. In another study treated mice were injected with human breast or colon cancer cells to induce cancer. The mice treated with modified citrus pectin had significantly less cancer spread to other areas than non-treated mice.[52]

A small pilot study presented at the international conference on diet and prevention of cancer, reported that five men out of seven tested had more than 30 percent lengthening of PSA doubling time when treated with modified citrus pectin.[53] Another, more recent study noted a similar increase in PSA doubling time in ten men out of a group of thirteen.[54] This increase was measured one year after the men began taking the citrus pectin and compared to their values before taking it. Keep in mind that these studies were of men who had already been diagnosed with recurrent prostate cancer. In men treated conventionally for prostate cancer, PSA levels are traditionally used as a marker for recurrence or metastasis. An increase in the amount of time it takes PSA to double in a man with recurrent prostate cancer can indicate that tumor growth has slowed.

While there is no definitive evidence that citrus pectin can cure prostate cancer, there certainly is evidence that it may help. The studies used a commercial product of modified citrus pectin called PectaSol® at a dose of fifteen grams per day, divided into three equal doses.* Other manufacturers have similar products.

A word of caution: Prostate cancer is a life-threatening condition that should not be self-treated. If you have prostate cancer, consult your doctor before trying any alternative or natural products or treatments.

More About Synergy

Throughout this book, I have mentioned the synergistic properties of various nutrients. Using them together can significantly enhance their effects. Herbs like saw palmetto, pygeum, nettle, and gingko are known to be quite safe with almost no side effects. Also, beneficial foods like pumpkin seeds, flaxseeds, and garlic (see Chapter Seven) can work together in a synergistic way to improve the function of the prostate as well as overall body health. Studies confirm statistically significant improvements in treatment of prostate problems—particularly BPH and prostatitis—with their use. But the

---

* PectaSol is a registered trademark of EcoNugenics, Inc.

complete mechanism by which they work is not known. Some researchers have singled out beta-sitosterol as the active ingredient in many of these herbs and foods. This hypothesis, however, does not account for the differences that occur when these herbs are taken together. Granted, beta-sitosterol is an important active constituent, but it is likely not the only one. It is more feasible that the components of these herbs and foods act synergistically with each other and other nutritive agents. All of the herbs in this chapter can be used together for a synergistic effect, and you will often find supplements that combine several of them. Such supplements are fine as long as they contain an adequate amount of each herb.

Interestingly, some studies noted an increase in sexual function with the herbal agents. These sexual improvements are most likely a result of generally improved health of the prostate gland.

Herbs that are high in phytoestrogens and phytosterols, particularly beta-sitosterol have been shown to be effective agents in the treatment of prostate disorders. Most notably, they are quite effective for helping men with BPH and prostatitis, and can also have a positive effect on erectile dysfunction and prostate cancer. These herbs have been well studied, individually and in conjunction with each other, for their synergistic effects.

The main action of many of them appears to be an amelioration of BPH by inhibiting the 5-alpha-reductase and aromatase enzymes, which reduce overall levels of DHT and estrogen. Saw palmetto, pygeum, nettle, and flower pollen appear to have this main action. Pumpkin and flaxseeds, on the other hand, are an excellent source of zinc, lignans, and other nutrients, while gingko and garlic improve blood circulation. The combination of a group of herbs and foods can attack prostate problems from several different directions. Coupled with low side effects, their synergistic effects make them the preferred treatment for mild prostate dysfunction. Many studies demonstrate and support the long-term use of herbal agents as a first-line treatment for uncomplicated BPH.[55, 56, 57, 58, 59, 60, 61] All of the herbs in this chapter along with the foods in the previous chapter can be used together for a synergistic effect.

A Word of Caution

Conventional medical treatment for BPH often is the drugs, Finasteride (Proscar, Propecia), Dutasteride (Avodart, Duogen), or Tamsulosin (Flomax). Each has significant side effects. Finasteride and Dutasteride are 5-alpha-reductase inhibitors. Tamsulosin works via a different mechanism. The 5-alpha-reductase enzyme is also believed to be inhibited by saw palmetto, which has been shown to be as effective as Finasteride with fewer side effects.[62] Treatment with a combination of herbs can be as (or more) effective than with the drugs, and sexual and other side effects are typically minimal. Herbs like saw palmetto, pygeum, and nettle that have an inhibiting effect on 5-alpha-reductase (as do the drugs) can theoretically cause interference with drug treatments, particularly Finasteride and Dutasteride, so it is unwise to use herbs in combination with these drugs.

The well-known side effects of each of these drugs are a reduction in (or loss of) libido, as well as problems with delayed or disrupted ejaculation, inability to have an orgasm (anorgasmia), and increased impotence. In addition to the sexual issues, dizziness, vision problems, and gynecomastia (enlarged breasts) have also been reported. Finasteride can be absorbed through the skin and can cause birth defects in male children if a pregnant woman comes in contact with it. Recent studies have stated that Finasteride can reduce the risk of getting prostate cancer, and some doctors have been prescribing it for this purpose. However, the prevention aspect is dulled by the underreported detail that Finasteride also increases the risk of developing aggressive and potentially fatal prostate cancer.[63]

More Cautions: PC-SPES and PC-HOPE

PC-SPES is a mixture of eight herbs that was promoted from around 1996 to 2002. It was marketed as a herbal hormonal treatment that could help slow the growth of prostate cancer. In February 2002, the

FDA claimed it contained prescription drugs and removed it from the market. PC-HOPE, a mixture of the same herbs and two additional ones, replaced it.

There was conflicting news about PC-SPES along with much controversy. Several clinical reports in major journals showed it had beneficial effects and could slow prostate cancer growth. Basically, both products are a form of hormonal therapy, usually known as androgen deprivation therapy or ADT, where hormones like testosterone are depleted in the body. Androgen deprivation therapy is typically used to treat prostate cancer that has spread beyond the gland, and it usually works for only a limited time. Earlier, I have noted research that shows that low testosterone levels are a risk factor rather than a cause of prostate problems. While herbal ADT may help slow the progression of metastatic prostate cancer, my opinion is that it is useless for prevention. I strongly suggest you steer clear of these products unless your doctor specifically recommends them.

Summary

Many studies show a clear association between diets rich in plant nutrients and a decreased risk of prostate dysfunction. In this chapter, we have looked at some herbs that have been found to be beneficial for the prostate. Simply using a combination of them for six months or so will often alleviate many prostate problems.

In the next chapter, I discuss nutrients and herbs that have a history of helping to resolve sexual problems or enhance libido. This is not to say that the herbs listed above will not help with such problems—they will. Many men report an increase in sexual performance after taking only the items discussed here. However, there are other herbs and nutrients that specifically tend to increase libido as well as sexual ability. Unfortunately, many of them are not as well studied as the ones in this chapter. Their reported benefits are often documented only in anecdotal folklore, or in advertising literature and pseudoscientific studies prepared by those that sell them.

Chapter Nine

Supplements to Help Overcome Erectile Dysfunction

We have examined several herbs that can help with BPH and pro-statitis. Often, coaxing the prostate to a better level of health with those herbs is enough to restore libido and help resolve erectile dys-function. For some men, however, the problem is more intense and may need additional prodding.

As we have discussed, hormone balance is critical to overall prostate health as well as sexual function. Many of the herbs dis-cussed in this book work their magic by helping the body balance hormone levels that have gone astray. While there are other ways to balance your hormone levels (discussed in Chapter Ten), it is best to start with herbal and nutritional approaches, and if they do not resolve the problem completely, then move on to supplementation with natural hormones.

Unfortunately, in the area of sexual dysfunction, there is much misleading information. This is particularly true for informa-tion on the Internet where supplement sellers can reach many men, and make almost any claim they want with little or no proof of effi-cacy. As a result, many items sold today for prostate or sexual prob-lems have little basis for recommending them other than the claims of the manufacturer or his agent. On the other hand, some herbs and nutritional items have considerable historical and anecdotal evi-dence, and a growing number have clinical evidence supporting their benefits.

Supplement manufacturers are quick to exploit any positive link to their products, and the pharmaceutical industry is also quick to promote negative information for natural items. A person in the middle, trying to sift through all the conflicting information, has a tough task indeed. The number of studies done in the United States on herbal remedies is far behind the rest of the world, but the gap appears to be closing. Herbal remedies are becoming more popular in the United States, and as a result, they are gathering more attention from researchers. While much of the herbal world is still based on folklore and historical use, studies that are more clinical are being done on natural preparations. In addition some medical doctors are starting to realize the value of herbal remedies and prescribe them.

I urge the reader to keep in mind that claims made about products that enhance libido or improve sexual performance are often false, and some products may actually cause adverse effects. I will discuss items for which I could find a reasonable amount of scientific or historical evidence that they work. I also urge the reader to keep in mind that while the prostate has much to do with sexual performance, it is only one member of a complex chorus. Generally, good health is crucial for a man's sexual ability. When health starts to wane, be it prostate or overall health, deterioration in sexual performance is not far behind.

In this chapter, I discuss herbs and amino acids that have both clinical and anecdotal evidence that they can help increase libido and sexual ability. Keep in mind that everyone is different. What works for one person, may or may not work for another. In addition many of the items discussed here have multiple modes of operation. If you try one combination and get little or no results, try another. Experiment and be patient. It often takes a few weeks for the effects of natural items to be felt.

There are many ways to overcome ED other than with drugs. I have tried to cover as many of the well-known remedies as possible as well as some of the lesser-known ones. I have presented those with the most solid evidence of effectiveness first. Most of these items have few side effects of significance, and where I found reports of any, they are listed.

Chemicals Involved in an Erection

An erection is a complex event that requires the cooperation of many body systems. During sexual arousal a series of chemical signals are initiated to cause the vascular changes that produce and maintain an erection. As a man becomes aroused sexually, nerve signals cause an increase in a chemical called nitric oxide (NO) in the genital area. This is the primary agent that begins a cascade of chemical actions that then result in an erection. Without nitric oxide, it would be impossible to produce an erection.

Nitric oxide stimulates release of another chemical called cyclic guanine monophosphate (cGMP), which enables smooth muscles surrounding the penile arteries to relax. This allows an inflow of blood into the penis producing an erection. However, if this were the entire picture, all men would be walking around with permanent erections. For the body to control the erection process, a substance called Phosphodiesterase-5 (PDE-5) is produced to eliminate the erection when it is no longer needed. PDE-5 deactivates cGMP allowing blood to drain out of the penis back into the body, thus *deflating* the erection. As we have discussed before, the body is all about balance. When all these substances are in balance, a firm erection is produced on sexual arousal, and on completion of sexual activity, the erection promptly dissipates.

Impotence drugs like Viagra and its counterparts are PDE-5 inhibitors. Decreased PDE-5 results in less breakdown of cGMP in the local penile arteries, helping to produce a more powerful and longer lasting erection. One of the drawbacks to this is that all drugs—including impotence drugs—have side effects. Over-inhibiting PDE-5 with a drug can cause an erection that does not subside with loss of sexual arousal, and can last for many hours. This condition is called "Priapism." It can be quite painful and can cause permanent damage to the penis due to the lack of normal blood circulation. Often, the only way to resolve priapism is with emergency medical treatment—typically surgery on the penis to allow the trapped blood to be released.

Endothelial Dysfunction

This is a medical term that refers to the thin layer of specialized cells called the *endothelium* that lines the inside of all blood vessels in the body. This tissue is involved in many biological processes, including those that control the constriction or dilation of blood vessels. Dysfunction in this tissue is linked to several chronic conditions, including but not limited to, erectile dysfunction, heart disease, and atherosclerosis.[1] One of the main indicators of endothelial dysfunction is a diminished level of nitric oxide. As explained above, nitric oxide is critical for proper erectile function. Thus, any item that improves endothelial function can help reduce the severity of erectile dysfunction and many other problems. This includes herbal or nutritional supplements as well as good foods like walnuts, peanuts, or other seeds and nuts. (See Chapter Seven.)

The International Index of Erectile Function Test (IIEF or IIEF-5)

This test, consisting of five questions, has evolved to be the standard for determining the severity of erectile dysfunction. It is shown in Figure 1 on the next page. To take the test, add your score for each of the five questions. The maximum score is twenty-five, the minimum five. The higher your score, the less the degree of erectile dysfunction. Typically, men with erectile dysfunction have an average score of about eleven, while men without erectile dysfunction usually score over twenty.

I suggest you record your current score and then come back to this test in six months or so, after you have begun a supplementation program. You may be pleasantly surprised.

L-Arginine

L-Arginine (or arginine) is a semi-essential amino acid that is prevalent in virtually all protein-rich foods, particularly nuts, seeds, fish,

Over the past few months	1	2	3	4	5
How do you rate your confidence that you could get and keep an erection?	Very low	Low	Moderate	High	Very high
When you had erections with sexual stimulation, how often were your erections hard enough for penetration?	Never or almost never	Much less than half the time	About half the time	Much more than half the time	Almost always or always
During sexual intercourse, how often were you able to maintain your erection after you had penetrated (entered) your partner?	Never or almost never	Much less than half the time	About half the time	Much more than half the time	Almost always or always
During sexual intercourse how difficult was it to maintain your erection to the completion of intercourse?	Extremely difficult	Very difficult	Difficult	Slightly difficult	Not difficult
When you attempted sexual intercourse, how often was it satisfactory for you?	Never or almost never	Much less than half the time	About half the time	Much more than half the time	Almost always or always

FIGURE 1. International Index of Erectile Function Test

and beans. There are many amino acids required by the body. They are the building blocks of protein. An essential amino acid cannot be made by the body and thus must be supplied by the food you eat. Arginine, being semi-essential, can be made by the body but is also an important element in the diet. Other foods high in arginine are coconut, barley, cinnamon, and chocolate. It is a natural compound, without which overall health of the body is compromised. Arginine acts as an agent to help increase nitric oxide (NO) levels in the blood. It reacts with an enzyme called nitric oxide synthase (NOS), and oxygen to produce nitric oxide. This reaction produces both NO and citrulline, another important amino acid that is discussed in the next section.

There are several enzymes and amino acids—like ornithine and citrulline—that play various roles in production of nitric oxide. Many of them convert bidirectionally, and the interplay between them is quite complex and not totally understood.

Normally, nitric oxide is abundant in the body, but aging or poor diet can result in inadequate production.[2] Without sufficient nitric oxide levels, it is impossible for a man to have and sustain an erection. Men with decreased levels of nitric oxide almost always suffer from erectile dysfunction.[3, 4, 5, 6, 7]

Nitric oxide is the primary chemical that acts to relax and dilate the smooth muscle tissue of penile arteries thus allowing sufficient blood flow into the penis for an erection. By helping increase the body's levels of nitric oxide, arginine can often resolve problems with erectile dysfunction. Studies have shown that about three to six grams of arginine daily will restore erectile function for most men.[8] In a good, randomized, double-blind, placebo-controlled study of fifty men, approximately one-third of the men reported a significant subjective improvement in sexual function. The duration of this study was six weeks, and the arginine dosage was five grams per day divided into three equal doses. However, the study authors note that the positive response was limited to men who had low nitric oxide levels at the start of the study.[9] One small study (twenty-one men) of a combination product containing three grams of arginine, along with ginseng (200 mg), ginkgo (50 mg), and several other vitamins and minerals, reported that 88.9 percent of the participants improved their ability to maintain an erection during sexual intercourse after four weeks using the product. No significant side effects were reported.[10]

Arginine has also been shown to help increase blood circulation through arteries clogged with cholesterol.[11] It may help overcome some of the negative effects of such clogged arteries—an important consideration for ED problems, as well as for those with cardiac insufficiencies. One study noted an increase in exercise tolerance in men with cardiovascular disease when using supplemental arginine.[12] This is probably due to its ability to increase nitric oxide levels in the body.[13, 14] In addition, several studies have found supplemental arginine and citrulline helpful for reducing age-related heart damage, cholesterol levels, and systolic blood pressure in both animals and humans.[15, 16, 17, 18, 19]

There are some experts who recommend taking up to twelve grams of arginine one hour prior to sexual activity. However, I could not find any studies to confirm its use at this higher level although several studies used higher doses for conditions other than erectile dysfunction. You may want to try taking the entire dose one hour before sexual activity if the divided dosing schedule does not work for you. Arginine comes in both capsules and powdered form that can be mixed with fruit juice or water.

It may take a few weeks for the effects of arginine to be noticed. It should not be used if you are using Viagra (or any of the other impotence drugs) or if you are being treated for a heart condition. Also, arginine may only help if your nitric oxide levels are low to begin with. However, since it could be difficult to get your nitric oxide levels measured, arginine is worth a try, especially since it is naturally occurring in food, safe, and has many other health benefits. If there is no improvement after six to eight weeks, you can assume your nitric oxide levels are relatively good and stop taking it.

L-Citrulline

Citrulline is an amino acid that is an integral part of nitric oxide synthesis and strongly related to arginine. In many tissues of the body that produce nitric oxide, citrulline is converted to arginine. Thus, supplemental citrulline can increase the availability of arginine. Citrulline is first converted to an arginine precursor in the liver, which is then used to convert citrulline to arginine in the endothelial tissue to produce nitric oxide.[20, 21] As discussed earlier in this chapter, dysfunction in this tissue due to aging is a primary cause of erectile problems. Citrulline is also produced by intestinal tissue and released into the bloodstream where it is converted to arginine by the kidneys. One study noted that significant quantities of arginine are synthesized in the kidneys from citrulline absorbed or produced in the intestines, and that the rate of arginine synthesis is independent of dietary arginine intake.[22] Another study noted significant increases in arginine and nitric oxide availability with supplemental citrulline at a rate of approximately 0.1 g/kg of body weight daily divided into two doses. This represents a dose of about eight grams per day for a 180-pound man.[23]

The availability of arginine depends in part on the concentration of other amino acids in the body. Oral supplementation with citrulline, as an amino acid precursor to arginine, can raise blood levels of arginine, and subsequently increase total available nitric oxide, greatly enhancing the potential for a normal erection in a man with erectile dysfunction. In addition, supplementation with both arginine and citrulline can help reduce many age-related problems with circulation.

A Word of Caution

In the studies reviewed no adverse effects were noted with either arginine or citrulline supplementation. However, they should not be used if you are taking any of the erectile dysfunction drugs. Viagra has been noted to increase the possibility of epileptic seizures in animals when taken in conjunction with arginine.[24] (See also *Viagra and its Cousins* in Chapter Five.) In addition, if you are being treated for a heart condition, you should consult with your doctor before using arginine or citrulline. You should also avoid foods and supplements containing high amounts of arginine if you have kidney disease or herpes simplex. High arginine levels can exacerbate both of these conditions. Protein-rich foods like most nuts, seeds, milk products, animal meat, seafood, and many legumes are high in arginine.

Arginine and Pycnogenol

Pycnogenol is a bioflavanoid extracted from various trees in the pine family and in grape seeds. The extract was patented around the mid-1980s. It is sold in most health food stores and on many websites. Some websites promote it as an aid to producing better erections. Nearly all the studies I found on this substance were several decades old, and done around the same time as the patent was granted. The only study related to erectile function used pycnogenol in conjunction with arginine. It noted an improvement in erectile function when pycnogenol was added to arginine. However, pycnogenol was not added until after one month of arginine supplementation, and that is when improved erectile function was noted.[25] In my opinion, the arginine supplementation (which typically takes about four to six weeks before results are seen), is more likely the item that produced the positive result. Simply getting a patent on a substance does not automatically confer it has any beneficial characteristics.

Yohimbe (Pausinystalia johimbe)

One of the most studied herbs for erectile dysfunction is Yohimbe. It comes from the Pausinystalia johimbe tree that is native to tropical West Africa. Its active ingredient is an alkaloid extracted from the bark known as yohimbine hydrochloride, or yohimbine. It was the first item approved for use by the FDA for erectile dysfunction. Yohimbine is available only as a prescription medicine. Standard extracts of the bark, however, also contain yohimbine and are available in health food stores.

Yohimbe's action is similar to other erectile dysfunction drugs currently available by prescription. It increases blood flow to the erectile tissue of the penis. Yohimbe differs from other impotence drugs in that it also tends to increase testosterone levels and thereby libido. In a double-blind study, yohimbe was given to eighty-two impotent men at a veteran's hospital. A 34 percent positive response was noted with only a few minor side effects.[26] Considering that the men in this population had a high incidence of diabetes and pathological vascular conditions, this is a remarkable result. Other studies have confirmed that yohimbe is effective for reducing erectile dysfunction in up to 55 percent of men.[27, 28, 29] This level of effectiveness is somewhat lower than that of other erectile dysfunction drugs. However, considering that yohimbe is a natural rather than synthetic agent, and also tends to increase libido, possibly via an increase in testosterone levels, it is worthwhile to consider it as a first-line treatment, especially for men with less severe problems.

There has been some question as to the safety of yohimbe when used directly from the bark, and some books have cautioned of dangerous side effects.[30, 31, 32] The most serious side effects the studies noted were a slight elevation of blood pressure and anxiety levels in some men. Other side effects appear to be minimal. If you are in the percentile of men for whom yohimbe is effective, you probably will not suffer any significant side effects. However, if you are prone to have high blood pressure, or you suffer from serious depression, panic attacks or anxiety, it is wise not to use yohimbe, since it could make such problems worse.

A word of caution—the extract yohimbine is the active ingredient of yohimbe bark. All of the studies referenced here used the prescription drug, yohimbine, for testing. The actual amount of yohimbine and potency of an extract depends on how the yohimbe bark is processed, and also on the manufacturer's integrity. One study of commercial yohimbe supplements found that many contain little or no yohimbine.[33] If you are going to try it, I suggest you stick to a well-known manufacturer's product, and stay away from supplements that advertise muscle or penile size gain.* Most manufacturers include some yohimbe in their male sexual enhancement products along with other items discussed in this chapter and Chapter Eight. Look for a supplement that contains a standardized extract of yohimbe bark yielding at least two, but no more than ten mg of yohimbines.

---

* To the best of my knowledge, there are no supplements that can increase penile size, but there is certainly no lack of advertisements to that effect.

Muria puama or Potency wood (Ptychopetalum olacoides)

This shrub is native to Brazil and is considered to be a powerful aphrodisiac and nerve stimulant in South American folk medicine. Both its leaves and roots are used medicinally. Muria puama has a long history. There are clinical studies on it going back as far as 1921 but few recent studies. The *British Herbal Pharmacopoeia,* a publication on herbal medicine from the British Herbal Medicine Association, has listed it as an herb for the treatment of sexual asthenia.* It is also listed in the *Brazilian Pharmacopeia of Herbal Medicine* for treatment of impotence.

One recent study of muria puama reported on 262 men with various degrees of erectile dysfunction and lack of libido. They were given between 1 and 1.5 grams per day of the herb.[34] Only minor side effects were noted. This study reported that 62 percent of the participants with low libido found it of benefit and 51 percent of those with erectile dysfunction were helped. Most participants noted positive effects within two weeks of starting treatment. A more recent study by the same author had similar results.[35]

While the mechanism of action of muria puama is unknown, the herb is highly regarded by herbalists worldwide, considered to be quite safe, and has substantial historical evidence supporting it. The referenced study claims it may be better than yohimbe at reducing the problems of sexual and erectile dysfunction. In my opinion, it is certainly worth a try for a few weeks at the dosage listed in the study. Again, as with most herbs, buy from a reputable manufacturer and purchase a standardized extract.

Ginseng (Panax ginseng)

Ginseng is an Asian herb with an extensive reputation as an aphrodisiac and sexual tonic. It is one of the most studied herbs for its

---

* Sexual asthenia is an older term typically replaced today by ED, impotence, or sexual dysfunction. Asthenia generally means lack of strength, weakness or debility.

other properties as well. Studies have shown it to be effective in modulating blood pressure, enhancing immune response, raising libido, and generally helping improve health. This reputation is well deserved. There are three different varieties (Asian: red panax ginseng; American: panax quinquefolius; and Siberian: eleutherococcus senticosus); that are commonly called Ginseng. While they have some similar properties, the Asian (sometimes called Korean) red panax ginseng has the most significant value for men with sexual dysfunction.

Panax ginseng has been shown in several studies of both animals and humans to promote increased sperm production, raise testosterone levels, and enhance erectile capacity.[36, 37] There is also some anecdotal evidence that it lowers the orgasmic threshold, making it easier for one to have an orgasm during sex. One study noted that it reduced the overall weight of the prostate gland in male rats after sixty days of use.[38] Other studies strongly suggest that ginseng may help raise HDL levels, while reducing total cholesterol levels. It is considered to be quite safe, and is often used as a geriatric tonic. A recent study specifically designed to measure toxicity concluded it has no measurable long-term toxic effects.[39]

There has been much written that people with hypertension should avoid Ginseng. Western medicine has long maintained that ginseng can cause serious side effects, including hypertension. Certain components of ginseng—called ginsenosides—have some effects that can be contradictory. As is typical with medicinal herbs, one element may balance or cancel the effects of another. This may account for the confusion. Some of ginsenosides in ginseng may cause some users to experience an increase in blood pressure and others to experience a decrease.[40] Generally, the evidence suggests that the effect of ginseng on blood pressure is to moderate it, hence the classification of ginseng as an adaptogen.*

In Asia, ginseng has enjoyed a positive reputation for people with cancer. Several recent reports have found that this reputation is

---

* An adaptogen is an herb that helps the body deal with various kinds of stress by normalizing body processes without adverse effects.

also well deserved. Some of the newly discovered ginsenosides in ginseng promote cancer cell death by selectively elevating protein levels of the p53 and other anti-cancer genes.[41, 42, 43] As we discussed in Chapter Three, the p53 gene plays an important role in initiating apoptosis of cancer cells. Other studies have found that ginseng has potent stimulating effects on the human immune system and that it confers significant protection from various cancers in both animals and humans.[44, 45, 46]

Ginseng does not have as strong an effect on erectile dysfunction as yohimbe or muira puama. Its main effect appears to be due to its influence on related systems. There is much science that proves this herb is quite valuable for balancing the body. It appears to affect many conditions, including prostate problems, cancer, sexual dysfunction, impotence, cholesterol and testosterone levels, and others.

Since ginseng can act as a stimulant, some users may notice side effects. Most notably, these are sleep problems or anxiety, and with higher doses, occasional heart palpitations. So, if you are being treated for a heart problem, you should be very cautious of ginseng. Also, a recent study confirmed a belief of several medical practitioners that ginseng reduces the effectiveness of blood thinning medication.[47] Users of any kind of prescription blood thinner (like Coumadin or Warfarin) should avoid ginseng supplements.*

When purchasing ginseng, select only Korean (Asian) red ginseng root extract standardized to provide 5 percent ginsenosides. Typical capsule sizes available vary from 100 to 400 mg. Keep in mind that individuals may respond differently to ginseng. It may work well for one person, but another might experience side effects. It is best to start with a low dose and watch for adverse effects. Typical dosage is about 300 to 1000 mg per day, but many individuals use more. Research studies have used up to 4,500 mg per day in test subjects without ill effects. Doses higher than typical should be used only under the direction of a health professional. Aside from the stated side effects, ginseng is generally considered to be a safe nontoxic herb.

*The study only looked at American Ginseng, but it is prudent to avoid all ginseng products if you are taking blood thinners.

Maca (Lepidium meyenii, Lepidium peruvianum)

Maca is an annual plant that is native to Peru. It is a cruciferous vegetable that produces a root similar to a turnip or potato and is a staple and versatile food product. Peruvians use it as Americans use potatoes and also to make cookies, cakes, chips, and various flavored drinks. Maca is an important food in the Peruvian diet with a rich nutrient profile. It grows in the Andes Mountains of Peru's Junin Plateau at elevations exceeding 10,000 feet.

Maca's reputation comes from a history of folklore of several hundred years. The Peruvian Inca people regarded it as an herb that can increase strength and stamina, as well as libido and sexual function. Today, Peruvian maca is still in high regard for its sexual enhancing abilities and it is cultivated and shipped worldwide for use in supplements.

Most of the supplements in this chapter have a direct effect on the mechanism that produces an erection. They either increase the chemical messengers that produce an erection or decrease those that prevent it. For some, the messenger is nitric oxide. For others, it is androgen hormones like testosterone. Maca is a notable exception. Clinical studies have shown that maca has virtually no effect on testosterone and the other sex steroid hormones.[48] It also does not appear to have any effect on nitric oxide levels. However, there are several good studies that agree the herb acts as an aphrodisiac, increasing sexual desire and ability. And it does all of this without affecting a man's hormone profile. While the studies show a positive effect, the mechanism for how it works is not clear.

There are many recent clinical studies on maca in both animals and adult men. All seem to agree that the herb increases sexual drive and ability. In animal studies, rats fed maca at about 75 mg per day per kilogram of their weight,* were observed to have a significantly greater sexual response.[49, 50, 51] I could find only one study of maca that looked for the same kind of enhanced sexual response in adult healthy men. This study did show a substantial improvement in

---

* This dose level is equivalent to about 5000 mg per day for a 150 lb. man.

sexual satisfaction after using maca and an increase in sexual desire and performance was seen after eight weeks of use.[52] Both animal and human tests have indicated maca stimulates the testis and increases production of sperm.[53, 54] While this may have nothing to do with erectile function, it may be an indicator that maca is helping to improve the health and strength of the entire genital system.

As a food, maca is loaded with nutrients. It is quite possible its reported benefits are due to its high concentration of protein, amino acids, phytosterols, and other nutrients. One recent study identified two previously unknown plant alkaloids in maca.[55] Maca is also high in arginine, phenylalanine, and histidine, all of which are essential amino acids and play different, but complementary, roles in sexual functioning. This high amino acid content of maca contributes to a protein level of about 10 percent. As discussed above, arginine is essential for production of the nitric oxide needed for an erection. Phenylalanine is also needed for proper nitrogen balance in humans and is converted in the body to tyrosine—a precursor for the hormones epinephrine, thyroxine, and others. Histidine is essential for the development and repair of tissues and is converted to histamine in the body. You may be familiar with histamine from its effect with allergic reactions, but you may not be aware that it also plays an important role in sexual performance. Histamine causes dilation of blood vessels and capillaries, helps constrict smooth muscle, and is ultimately a primary player in ejaculation and orgasm. Although maca generally has a high amino acid content, it is relatively low in the amino acid methionine, which, coincidentally, is a strong antihistamine. Thus, this unique combination of amino acids and other nutrients might be what gives maca its reputed powers.

A word of caution: maca has often been touted as a natural answer to Viagra. Maca suppliers and others with financial interests in it have funded some of the research referenced above. Since maca is a known food staple with a fabulous nutrient profile, it is unlikely that it will do any harm other than to your wallet. Considering that it is relatively inexpensive and safe, I believe it is certainly worth a try. Buying maca in capsules, however, is not going to be effective. Peruvians eat considerable amounts of maca as a vegetable staple on a routine basis, so a few hundred milligrams of dried root in a capsule is unlikely to have any effect. The best way to buy it would be as a bulk, powdered herb, or as the complete root in a health food store. You can use the powder in a beverage, or cook and eat the root as you would a potato or a turnip. There does not seem to be any toxicity or adverse effects to using maca, even in large doses.

Horny Goat Weed – (Epimedium grandiflorum or Epimedium sagittatum)

The popular name of this herb alone might make a man with ED want to buy it. But aside from the provocative name, horny goat weed has a reputation that stretches back more than 2000 years. In Chinese medicine, it is known as Yin Yang Huo. The legend is that ancient Chinese goat herders noticed their animals becoming more sexually active after grazing on this weed, hence the name. Its traditional use is for treating disorders of the kidneys and liver as well as sexual dysfunction. Most of the research done on this herb comes from China, where it has been studied for many years.

Epimedium is a slow growing, creeping perennial plant with semievergreen leaves that grows primarily in China. It is often used decoratively for ground cover. Epimedium has a long history of use to improve erectile function and libido in the folklore of many cultures. The parts of the plant used medicinally are its leaves, which contain a variety of plant sterols, flavonoids, polysaccharides, and alkaloids. The most active component of horny goat weed is believed to be a compound called icariin.

Its reputation for increasing libido has been noted in several studies, but there are many theories as to how horny goat weed works. Chinese herbalists believe it helps the body restore levels of testosterone—particularly free testosterone—and thyroid hormones. This effect was noted in an animal study and may be due to various testosterone-like components of the plant's leaves.[56]

Horny goat weed also appears to cause blood vessels and capillaries to dilate, thus increasing blood flow to the sexual organs. One study was done on mice with erectile dysfunction induced by poor arterial circulation. The study concluded that epimedium significantly improved erectile function and nitric oxide levels in the erectile tissue of the tested mice.[57]

A credible Chinese study investigated the effects of horny goat weed on twelve patients with chronic kidney disease. The study concluded that it had a significant positive effect on sexual dysfunction and helped increase the immune function in these patients.[58] Another study noted a statistically significant protective effect on the immune system for patients taking steroid medications.[59] Such medications, called glucocorticoids, typically have the effect of suppressing immune response and adrenal function. While this is not directly related to erectile function, it does confirm the immune enhancing functions of horny goat weed reported in other studies.[60]

Most studies of epimedium have been primarily related to its use in Chinese medicine. While the Chinese do use it as an aphrodisiac, it has been studied more for its use for treating chronic kidney and liver problems, osteoporosis, and enhancing immunity. There are few clinical reports supporting its use for erectile dysfunction or libido problems. At the time of this writing, however, a search of the Internet for "horny goat weed" brings up more than two million sites, most of them extolling a multitude of virtues for this herb. Of course, nearly all of these sites are selling commercial epimedium products. In some cases, clinical studies are cited for the products, but such studies—almost always financed by the manufacturer—often stretch the scientific evidence far beyond reality. That said, the folklore for horny goat weed is impressive, and I did not find any reports of adverse effects associated with its use at the recommended dosage. Based on the folklore and its relative safety, it may be worth a try.

The most frequently marketed epimedium products are usually extracts standardized to contain at least 10 percent icariin. It is interesting to note that the herb contains several different active compounds. The standard use in Chinese medicine is to brew the leaves in hot water as a tea. Taking the herb this way results in a broad profile of its many active components. Unfortunately, to use it this way you need to buy the herb in bulk and brew it yourself. While this is probably the most effective way to use this herb, it may also be the most inconvenient. A typical dose of an extract is 500 mg twice daily. Some manufacturers add some ground leaf to the product. This may be a good compromise, as the extract yields a standardized icariin content, and the whole leaf provides other active constituents.

Tribulus or Puncture vine (Tribulus terrestris)

Tribulus is a tropical perennial shrub in the bean-caper family that grows in warm, arid regions. It has been used for hundreds of years as a treatment for both male and female sexual problems and has a reputation among bodybuilders for building muscle. In many countries it is widely used by athletes. In India, tribulus is used in ayurveda, the ancient Hindu science of health and medicine, as both a tonic and aphrodisiac. Rumor has it that it is used by many top eastern European weightlifters.

The promotion of tribulus is primarily as a testosterone booster, hence its reputation for building muscle. However, while the body-building sites extol its virtues, clinical studies have not been so kind. One study designed to determine the effects of tribulus on weightlifters found that supplementation with tribulus did not enhance body composition or exercise performance.[61] In fact, at the end of this study, men untreated with tribulus showed greater gains in endurance than the treated group.

Tribulus does, however, seem to enhance libido. It appears to increase testosterone by a different path then hormonal precursors like DHEA and androstenedione. (See Chapters Three and Ten.) According to some studies, tribulus increases production of luteinizing hormone (LH) in the pituitary gland. Luteinizing hormone is the chemical messenger that stimulates cells in the testicles to produce testosterone. An increase in LH will generally cause a corresponding rise in testosterone levels. Some sources say that tribulus increases LH levels by more than 70 percent and free testosterone levels by more than 40 percent, but I could find no clinical confirmation of this. Studies seem to agree that while tribulus does raise testosterone levels, the effect is more pronounced on men that already have low levels. There is some evidence that tribulus increases levels of DHEA and androstenedione, but it is not clinically proven.

While there is an abundance of information about tribulus on the Internet, few studies have been published in respected medical journals. Manufacturers of tribulus supplements author most available reports and thus they are typically biased towards their products. One manufacturer's study, whose results were reviewed by several prominent researchers in Bulgaria, found that twelve of fourteen patients with reduced libido (treated with tribulus for thirty days) showed an obvious improvement in sexual desire. In addition, out of thirty-six patients with prostatitis and low libido, twenty-seven noted improvement in symptoms. This study also noted an increase in luteinizing hormone, and an increase in testosterone levels, particularly in the men whose levels were low before treatment.[62] Again, keep in mind that a manufacturer of a tribulus product sponsored this study, and it has not been published in any medical journal. However, animal studies appear to support its results.[63] One animal study noted a decrease in blood pressure in hypertensive rats fed tribulus.[64]

In its favor, tribulus contains phyto-chemicals called steroidal furostanol saponins, or more simply saponins. One of them, called "protodioscin" is known to improve sexual desire and enhance erection. Studies in animals and humans have shown that protodioscin increases levels of both testosterone and DHEA.[65, 66] Other saponins also appear to be active in tribulus and may account for some of its activity. Tribulus is a complex herb that seems to have interesting effects on the body. New saponins recently discovered may be found to be as, or more active, than protodioscin regarding libido enhancement or erectile function.[67, 68]

Unfortunately, the amount of these active agents may vary considerably between plants grown in differing soils. To get significant amounts of the saponins the plant must be harvested at the right time of year and properly stored and processed. A recent study noted significant differences ranging from 0.17 to 6.49 percent in protodioscin content in various commercial products.[69] This may account for the different results in some of the studies.

There are no reported problems with using tribulus, and it does not appear to have any serious side effects. Even so, tribulus has been known to have toxic effects on sheep. If you decide to try it, start with a low dose and gradually increase it watching for any adverse effects. Purchase only an extract from a reputable manufacturer, standardized to contain at least 20 percent protodioscin, and a minimum of 30 to 40 percent steroidal saponins (furostanol). A typical dosage is 750-1500 mg daily, divided into three doses at mealtimes.

Cnidium, Monier's Snowparsley, Shi Chuang Zi (Cnidium monnieri)

Another herb that grows in Asia, cnidium, is finding use in sexual enhancement products worldwide. It has been widely used in China for more than a thousand years as a treatment for impotence, and for a variety of skin and liver ailments. In traditional Chinese medicine, cnidium is known as Shi Chuang Zi. Its use in the United States is almost exclusively as an ingredient in male sexual enhancement formulas.

Several studies have shown cnidium to be effective in relaxing the smooth muscle tissue of the corpus cavernosa in animals. Relaxing this tissue is part of the process of obtaining an erection in both animals and humans. The studies found that the group of plant compounds called coumarins in cnidium are effective in causing a release of nitric oxide, a corresponding increase in cGMP (cyclic guanine monophosphate) and a decrease in the erection killing phosphodiesterase-5 (PDE-5). One coumarin in particular, called osthole, was found to significantly increase levels of cGMP.[70] As discussed at the beginning of this chapter, cGMP is the substance that helps relax smooth muscle tissue and produce an erection. On the other hand, PDE-5 digests cGMP, eliminating its effect and the erection. Other animal studies indicate cnidium is a potent PDE-5 inhibitor.[71, 72] Prescription impotence drugs like Viagra work their magic by inhibiting PDE-5. Thus, cnidium has the potential to have a significant effect on erectile dysfunction by the same pathways as the prescription drugs—inhibiting PDE-5. Cnidium may have the additional advantage of increasing cGMP.

Since there are no human studies available, I could not find any specific dosing information for cnidium. Also, it is not generally available as a single herb, but is more often packaged as one component of a multiple ingredient male enhancement formula. If you do want to try it, stick with a product from a reputable manufacturer and follow their instructions.

Tongkat ali, Eurycoma, or Longjack (Eurycoma longifolia Jack)

Tongkat ali, or Eurycoma, is a medium-sized tree that grows up to forty-five feet high. It is native to Southeast Asia and ubiquitous in Malaysia. This herb has recently been introduced into the United States, but it has a long history of medicinal use in Asia. All parts of the plant are used medicinally. While its primary use in Asia is as an aphrodisiac, it also has many other folk uses. Traditional Malaysian folk medicine practitioners use it to treat malaria, eliminate parasites, and to treat cancerous tumors, particularly those of the lung and breast. There is scientific evidence that the historical folk use is on target.[73, 74, 75]

Folklore has it that tongkat ali increases libido by increasing testosterone, hence it is an ingredient in some bodybuilding formulas. However, since there does not seem to be any human studies, it is impossible to verify or disprove this claim. Several studies appear to confirm its ability to improve sexual drive and performance in animals. At the University of Science, School of Pharmaceutical Sciences in Malaysia, a group of researchers confirmed the ability of tongkat ali to increase libido of mice and rats.[76, 77, 78, 79, 80, 81] Unfortunately, there does not appear to be any similar studies in men. The dosage used in these studies was escalated from 200 to 800 milligrams per kilogram of body weight, with sexual behavior of the animals increasing proportional to the dosage. This dose rate for a man weighing approximately 160 pounds translates to between 15 and 60 grams per day of the whole herb. Since this is a rather large amount to consume, tongkat ali is usually sold as a 100:1 concentrated extract. This brings a typical dose to 145 mg/day and the escalated dose to 580 mg/day. With a typical product containing 80 mg of 100:1 extract, you could start with two tablets daily. If no effects are felt after three to four weeks, increase the dosage to four tablets per day. Unfortunately, since it takes a lot of raw herb to make an extract, and all tongkat ali sold in this country is imported, it is rather expensive. A typical retail price for a month's supply is about fifty dollars.

While there are no clinical studies done with eurycoma on humans, there is a substantial amount of anecdotal evidence and testimonials associated with it. Most men who try it report a noticeable and substantial increase in libido. Another indicator that the plant may be of significant value as an aphrodisiac is that an Indonesian pharmaceutical company is studying it, and both Japanese and European companies have applied for patents for sexual enhancement products made from it.

The only way eurycoma is useful is as a standardized extract of at least 100:1. Whole herb supplements or extracts of less than 100:1 are not likely to provide enough of the active constituents to cause any effect. I could not find any reports of adverse reactions.

Oats (Avena sativa)

Avena sativa, also called "wild oats" or "oats," is a tall annual grass, about three to four feet high, that grows wild in temperate and subtropical climates. Historically, oat grain was widely used for making breakfast cereals, but this application has declined with the increased availability of wheat grains. Avena has a mild, creamy flavor and is probably best known for its use in breakfast cereals. However, both seed and grain can be used in other ways. Oatmeal is a popular and nutritious food, well suited for individuals with stomach problems. Ground oat seed is historically used as a poultice for the treatment of dry skin and eczema.

While avena has been used mainly as food, there is significant research confirming its medicinal value. It is extremely nutritious and has a broad nutrient profile. Regular consumption can increase stamina and generally help in recovering from debilitating illnesses. Consumption of a diet rich in oat bran has been proven to lower cholesterol levels in the blood. Oats are also high in beta-sitosterol, which (as discussed in Chapter Eight), is a known nutrient that supports prostate health.

There is considerable information about avena sativa on the Internet, much of it related to improving sex drive. Legend has it that farmers observed their stallions getting sexually active after eating wild oat grain, hence the reputation. Rare is the person that has not heard the expression "sowing his oats," referring to a young man's sexual activity.

Unfortunately, those who are selling avena supplements for libido improvement have generated nearly all the available information. In fact, most of its sex-boosting claims are from research done by a single group that markets avena products. These promoters say that avena releases testosterone bound to SHBG, thus increasing free testosterone levels. Of course, if it did increase free testosterone levels it would surely have an effect on libido. There is little scientific basis for this effect, however, and I could find no clinical research that supports this claim.

On the other hand, there is a considerable amount of research proving that a regular diet including avena (as oatmeal) can lower cholesterol levels considerably.[82, 83, 84] And lowering cholesterol can improve blood flow throughout the body and lower blood pressure, both of which can help reduce erectile dysfunction.

Oatmeal contains lots of fiber, and as I mentioned above, it has a rich nutrient profile. At the beginning of this chapter I discussed the effects of arginine on erectile performance. One hundred grams of oat grain, in a bowl of breakfast cereal supplies more than one gram of arginine along with a host of other amino acids and nutrients. It is certainly possible that a diet high in oat grain could increase sexual performance simply by the reduction of cholesterol deposits in one's arteries, along with the increased nitric oxide stimulated by the high arginine content. While avena sativa cannot truly be called a sexual enhancement supplement, it certainly can help improve your overall health. If you do want to try an extract, purchase one standardized to contain at least 10 percent steroidal avenacosides. Typical dosage is 100-200 mg per day. Many supplements combine avena sativa with tribulus terrestris to enhance the effect. However, I suspect the tribulus, which has proven ability to raise testosterone levels, is the more active constituent. If you want to try adding this to your health regimen, I recommend you add it as a food like oatmeal. Most supplements, even extracts, contain too little avena to actually be useful.

Red kwao krua (Butea superba)

Butea is a member of flowering plants belonging to the pea family. It is native to India, Thailand, and other Southeast Asian areas. Its many species are used for resins, dyes, and medicine. Butea superba, the species abundantly distributed in Thai deciduous forests, is traditionally used in herbal preparations as a male aphrodisiac.

Considerable research exists for this herb regarding its chemical composition. Butea has a relatively high antioxidant content, along with a level of plant chemicals resembling human androgens.[85] There is little scientific evidence supporting its use for erectile dysfunction other than folklore and one human study. However, it is used in traditional Thai medicine as a major ingredient in herbal mixtures for the treatment of erectile dysfunction and rejuvenation of sexual vigor. Some supplement manufacturers claim that butea superba has some anticholinesterase activity. This would imply that it would increase levels of acetylcholine, a known mediator of erectile function as well as memory. But the only information I could find to support this claim was on another species of butea, not the butea superba species used in the supplement.

It is believed that butea inhibits the enzyme PDE-5 in the same way as cnidium (described above). As previously discussed, inhibiting PDE-5 aids in dilation of blood vessels in the penis and adds to the quality of an erection. The one study I did find was a randomized, double-blind clinical trial of thirty-nine Thai males, ranging in age from thirty to seventy, with various degrees of sexual dysfunction.[86] They were given 800 mg per day of butea in divided doses over a three-month period. The study concluded that 82 percent of them showed some improvement, and 36 percent reported an excellent response at the end of the study period. No evidence of toxicity was reported. Since this herb seems to have actions similar to cnidium, it may have a similar effect on erectile dysfunction, but more studies on it would be welcome.

Xanthoparmelia Scabrosa

This ingredient of a few sexual enhancement products is a lichen rather than an herb. Lichens are symbiotic organisms made from the association of microscopic algae and fungus. They typically grow on rocks and tree trunks, forming a crust-like growth on the surface. This particular lichen is found throughout Asia, Australia, and South America. Lichens have many chemicals in them that could have profound effects on the human body. The only clinical studies I could find on this lichen note that some of its components have shown antitumor activity against human cancer cell lines in the laboratory.[87, 88]

There is little clinical information available for xanthoparmelia scabrosa and no human studies. One manufacturer of a sexual stimulant claims that its extract of xanthoparmelia scabrosa called "Xantho-Pure" has been proven very effective as a PDE-5 inhibitor. While the manufacturer's literature is convincing, I could not find any scientific evidence to support the claim. Additionally, in a 2004 newsletter, the American Society of Pharmacognosy repeated a warning from the National Nutritional Foods Association—Midwest Region (NNFA-MW), that xanthoparmelia scabrosa has been shown to contain a toxic ester that can damage cells. According to the NNFA-MW, both the FDA and the FTC are aware of this possible toxicity. I recommend you avoid sexual enhancement products that contain this herb until this matter is defined more clearly.

Other Herbs Used in Commercial Products

There are many herbs I could list in this chapter that are commonly used in male sexual enhancement products. Unfortunately, most of them have little scientific basis for their use. While (in some cases) the folklore is strong, I have limited this chapter to a discussion of herbs that have some clinical data in addition to anecdotal evidence or folklore. This is not to say that some of these commercial products are useless, but just that there is not much data supporting them. Some have a long history of safe use and could indeed be of some value for prostate or sexual healing. For example, the herb sarsaparilla is used in many sexual enhancement products because of the natural, testosterone-like, substances it contains. The claim is that the herb increases available testosterone in the body. Whether or not the substances in sarsaparilla have any effect on testosterone levels is unknown, but that does not stop many manufacturers from making the claim. Likewise, catuaba, another herb from the Amazon rain forest, has significant historical folklore touting its use as a sexual enhancer. It too is used in many prostate supplements. Again, the folklore on catuaba is strong, and perhaps there is some truth to it, but the only clinical study I could find was one that measured its effect on rabbit corpus cavernousm (penile erectile tissue). That study concluded that it had no effect.[89]

In many cases, other obscure herbs are used as part of herbal sexual enhancement or male health formulas in addition to one or more of the herbs detailed above that have actual clinical results supporting their efficacy. Again, this is not to say that these products are ineffective or useless, and indeed some of them may have an effect. But without further research, their usefulness, as well as their safety, remains unknown.

Synergy

I have mentioned synergy many times in this book. In a recent well-designed study, a combination of arginine and yohimbine was compared with yohimbine alone in a group of forty-five men.[90] The patients with mild to moderate ED responded better to the combination of arginine and yohimbe than to yohimbe alone, and both groups did better than a placebo group. This synergistic effect often occurs with other herbs and vitamins as well. You may find that a combination of one or more of the items discussed in this chapter taken together may be more helpful than any single item taken alone. Just be sure to start slow, adding only one item at a time, and be mindful of any side effects. Remember that herbal agents often work by enhancing overall health, and it may take several weeks to notice improvement.

Things to Avoid

In this chapter, I have discussed several nutrients and herbs that are beneficial for a man with ED. However, there are also some items that can worsen the situation.

Licorice — This herb, an ingredient in many candies, flavoring agents, breath fresheners, over-the-counter remedies, and even some male sexual enhancement products, can cause problems when consumed regularly or in large quantities. Licorice contains a chemical called glycyrrhizin that can deplete the body's potassium, cause water retention, and lead to high blood pressure. This can happen with as little as five to seven grams of licorice root per day on a regular basis. Of additional concern to a man with ED is that licorice has been reported to lower testosterone levels.[91] This is certainly not what a man suffering from ED wants. Licorice is also one of the ingredients in the herbal preparation PC-SPES mentioned in the previous chapter. One study found that as little as 500 mg of glycyrrhizin per day for one week (the amount in approximately 7 grams of licorice) significantly lowered serum testosterone levels in healthy men.[92] The study noted that testosterone levels fell by approximately 40 percent after four days of consuming the licorice.

On the other hand, another study concluded that decreases in testosterone levels due to the glycyrrhizin in licorice were not significant.[93] Differences between these studies may be due to how licorice affects testosterone levels in each individual. Some individuals may be more sensitive to its effects than others. Also, in the second study, hormones were measured in saliva rather than blood serum. Levels measured in saliva yield values for only free or unbound hormones (see Chapter Ten), and only free testosterone is active. This may also account for some of the different responses noted in the studies. Diabetic men, in particular, may suffer more from the effects of licorice than healthy men. One group of researchers in Japan, where licorice is used as a treatment for chronic hepatitis, studied the effects of licorice on a small group of diabetic men. They reported that serum concentrations of both total and free testosterone were significantly lower in the men consuming glycyrrhizin.[94]

If you currently consume licorice and you suffer from erectile dysfunction, it would be wise for you to curtail licorice consumption for several months to see if your symptoms improve. Fortunately, it appears that the effect licorice has on the body is reversed when consumption of it is eliminated. In any event, it is probably wise to avoid any more than occasional use of licorice, especially if you suffer from erectile dysfunction or hypertension.

Fatty Meals — As we noted earlier, high fat meals, particularly those high in animal fat, lead to many problems with the prostate and general health. Often a man will consume a large meal and later finds that an attempt at sexual intercourse results in failure.

When your body is busy digesting a heavy meal, it is not going to be able to divert a significant amount of blood from the digestion process to the penis. The solution is simple—eat a lighter meal or wait longer to digest a heavier one before attempting sexual activity.

Medications for Depression, High Blood Pressure, and Pain Relief — Many prescription drugs—particularly antidepressants—have a long history of causing sexual problems, both by reducing libido and causing erectile dysfunction. This is very well-known and has been documented in clinical studies. If you are on antidepressants and you suffer from erectile dysfunction, consult with your doctor about possibly switching to a different drug or using some of the herbs suggested in this book to offset the side effects. (See ginkgo in Chapter Eight.) Often, an herb like ginkgo may help to reduce the problem, but discuss it with your doctor first. Some of the newer drugs for these conditions have less sexual side effects.

In addition, some commonly used pain relievers, known as NSAIDs (nonsteroidal anti-inflammatory drugs) like ibuprofen or naproxen, as well as the prescription drug Celebrex, can have a profound effect on the prostate, causing irritation and/or urinary retention. In a Dutch study men who were actively using NSAIDs had double the risk of developing acute urinary retention.[95] It is well-known that several types of cold remedies containing antihistamines can cause severe prostate irritation, particularly when used by men with BPH.

Marijuana — While not generally as dangerous as some of the other illicit drugs, marijuana has produced controversial results when studied for its effects on sexual functioning. Some studies have shown it to lower testosterone and other androgen levels, particularly in older men.[96, 97, 98] Other studies have shown it to have little effect on testosterone levels.[99, 100] It is interesting to note that most of these studies were done decades ago. The current mind-set linking marijuana to more addictive and damaging drugs prevents many researchers from studying it. My opinion is that smoking marijuana can have a negative effect on sexual ability and cause erectile dysfunction, particularly in older men.

A recent article in a cardiology journal relates a case history of a young man having a heart attack after the recreational use of Viagra and marijuana.[101] Smoking marijuana can cause changes in heart rate and blood pressure, which can be dangerous, especially when combined with other drugs.

Marijuana smokers inhale carcinogens with the smoke just like tobacco smokers. A recent study implicated it as a causative factor for the same kind of cancers caused by tobacco.[102] Thus, it is prudent to avoid it. And most certainly, it is not a substance to be used in conjunction with an erectile dysfunction drug!

Other Illicit Drugs — Most of the other illicit drugs have a clear history of producing addiction and inhibiting sexual drive and ability. Some—like cocaine—produce an initial euphoria that may lead to heightened sexual performance for a short while. However, with continued use the euphoria fades, and sexual ability is crippled. Other drugs—like those in the opiate family (heroin, morphine, methadone, etc.), are central nervous system depressants and typically inhibit both sexual desire and ability almost immediately. With their continued use the effect tends to multiply, eventually resulting in an almost complete lack of libido and total or near total impotence. If you value your sex life, do not mess with illicit drugs!

Summary

Unfortunately, there is not a tremendous amount of controlled scientific studies on the effects of natural substances for erectile dysfunction. To compound the problem, much of the research done in this area has occurred outside of the United States, preventing widespread knowledge in this country due to language problems and inaccessibility of some publications. Fortunately, the Internet and popular search engines like Google have now matured to the point where such information is becoming readily available.

In this chapter I have covered much material and have discussed many items that can help increase your libido and reduce problems with erectile dysfunction. However, natural substances tend to work slowly, and may not work the same in all individuals. If, for example, low levels of nitric oxide are causing your erectile dysfunction, the amino acids arginine or citrulline may help. On the other hand, if your problem is low libido due to low testosterone levels, then supplemental amino acids will be of little value.

The ideal situation would be to test all pertinent items that effect sexual performance, and then take the appropriate substances to correct any problems. This would require a specialized clinic that treats erectile dysfunction. Such treatment is now becoming available, but it is expensive. The other drawback is that this type of care is rarely covered by insurance and is hard to find—even if your wallet can handle the costs.

In addition to nutritional or herbal items, many men have had good success using pelvic floor exercises (also known as Kegel exercises) to help overcome erectile dysfunction. It is beyond the scope of this book to explain these exercises, but an excellent discussion of them can be found in *The Testosterone Syndrome* by Eugene Shippen, M.D., listed in the bibliography.

If you try some of the herbs mentioned in this chapter, be patient. With many nutritional or herbal agents, it takes several weeks before their effects are felt. If one product does not work, try another, or try a compound product that has several of the herbs discussed here.

If you suspect your problem is hormonal, start with the herbs that tend to balance or raise testosterone levels like ginseng, tribulus, or yohimbe. A combination of one or more of these may help your body produce more testosterone and may resolve ED problems without further action. If there is no improvement after a month or two, you may want to have your hormone levels tested. Extremely low free testosterone levels may need to be restored to normal using bio-identical hormone cream. This is discussed in the next chapter.

Chapter Ten

Natural (Bio-Identical) Hormone Balancing

In Chapters Three and Four, we looked at the role hormones play in the development of prostate dysfunction. We also examined some lifestyle issues that cause them to get out of balance. As I pointed out, such hormone imbalances are often the result of many different factors and are often seen in studies of men that already have prostate dysfunction. In particular, low testosterone coupled with high estrogen levels can be an early indicator of impending prostate or sexual problems.

In this chapter, I discuss how to find out where your hormone levels are and how to balance them using natural or bio-identical hormones.* Much of this information comes from the work and writings of the late John R. Lee, M.D., who used natural hormones for many years in his medical practice and wrote several books on the subject. (See the bibliography.)

We have all heard of athletes using various hormones to boost their performance. Typically, these are known as anabolic steroids. Using such hormones to enhance performance is, at best, risky and at worst, seriously threatening to one's health. Performance enhancements gained this way are typically short-lived and come at a high price—often years later. Anabolic steroids are known to cause liver toxicity, testicular atrophy, breast enlargement, excessive cholesterol levels, erectile dysfunction, and other serious

---

* Bio-identical hormones are substances that are identical to those produced naturally by the body.

conditions. The only realistic goal for hormone supplementation is to restore your levels to their biological norms.

There is a popular misconception that men, unlike women, do not need hormone replacement as they age. Men typically do not have a specific point at which symptoms of hormone decline (sometimes called "andropause") appear. In most men, symptoms appear gradually and are not usually noticed until they become severe. A man may experience occasional erectile dysfunction due to imbalanced hormones and not become concerned until the occasional erection failure becomes the rule rather than the exception. Often his ED is accompanied by a lack of vigor, poor muscle tone, depression, and low energy—all symptoms of declining testosterone levels. Unfortunately, many men with such symptoms accept them as inevitable and never seek help.

As I discussed earlier, men begin to have slightly lowered levels of the sex steroid hormones as they enter their forties. These lowered hormone levels usually produce only minor symptoms, which are typically dismissed as inevitable consequences of aging. However, as a man progresses through his fifties, sixties, and seventies, such symptoms become more pressing. It is my belief that early hormone disturbances are precursors to more serious prostate dysfunction. Addressing these imbalances with good nutrition, herbal supplementation, and if warranted, hormone replacement, could prevent many problems.

A recent study of men with prostate cancer who were scheduled for surgical removal of their prostates, compared testosterone levels with the results of analysis of the excised tissue. Mean testosterone levels were significantly lower in the men with positive surgical margins in the removed gland.* Typically, this is considered a marker for aggressive disease that is difficult to manage. It is also interesting that testosterone levels for all men in this study was rather low, averaging 284.7 ng/dl for men in the aggressive cancer group,

---

*Positive surgical margins means that cancerous cells were found that extended beyond the portion of the tissue removed by the surgery.

and 385.7 ng/dl for the others.* The normal range of testosterone levels for men over sixty is approximately 350 to 720 ng/dl. In younger men the upper value is nearly twice as high. Remember, in this study all the men had prostate cancer, and even the men with less aggressive disease had relatively low testosterone levels. In my opinion the result of this study adds to the ever-increasing information suggesting that low testosterone levels are associated with prostate disease.[1] Another study was designed to compare androgen levels of men newly diagnosed with prostate cancer to a similar group of men with BPH. Again, the men with cancer were found to have significantly lower testosterone activity then the men with BPH. And the men with more aggressive cancer had even lower levels.[2]

As explained in earlier chapters, hormone imbalances in aging men are primarily the result of decreased testosterone and progesterone, and increased SHBG and estrogen. Subsequently, this results in an increase in the body's estrogen to testosterone ratio. Stimulation of receptors in the prostate via estrogens, along with lower levels of androgens, particularly testosterone, contribute significantly to the onset of BPH, erectile dysfunction, and prostate cancer.[3] Unfortunately, most men (including this author) wait too long before they admit that their early, minor symptoms have become significant. At that point it is harder to correct the problems. Thankfully, they are still correctable. To correct such imbalances, we need to increase the effective testosterone to estrogen ratio. This is done by increasing testosterone levels, reducing estrogen levels, or blocking some of the negative effects of the estrogens.

Determining Hormone Levels

There are many natural ways to recover from age-related hormonal imbalances. Earlier I discussed several herbs that can help. However, using herbs for this purpose can be hit or miss, especially

---

* ng/dl = nanogram per decaliter

if you do not know exactly which hormones are out of balance, or how far out they are. Supplementing with natural hormones can alleviate some of the age-related problems for most men over forty. But with the exception of using low doses of natural progesterone (see below), it is imperative that you test your hormone levels prior to supplementing. This is simple and can be done with a saliva test kit from any one of several testing laboratories. The appendix contains information on laboratories supplying such kits. You can purchase the kits directly from the laboratories or from my website. The kits are easy to use, requiring that you simply put a saliva sample in a tube and mail it to the testing laboratory.

Alternately, you can visit your medical practitioner and have a blood hormone profile taken. Unfortunately, most medical doctors only use blood tests and only order tests for total hormone concentration (see Chapter Three). It is common for older men to have a normal level of total testosterone, but low free testosterone. Since only the free component is active, measurement of total testosterone can be misleading. For the test to be meaningful, your doctor must specify measurement of both. According to many experts, saliva is better suited for measuring hormone levels than blood since saliva contains only free hormones.

At the very least, you should measure levels of free testosterone, DHT, progesterone, estradiol, and DHEA. In addition if you suffer from fatigue, depression, dry skin, dry hair, cold hands and feet, or you always tend to feel cold, or have significant problems losing weight, you may be suffering from hypothyroidism (low thyroid hormone levels). It is a simple matter for your doctor to test your thyroid hormone levels, and hypothyroidism is frequently associated with low testosterone levels and erectile dysfunction. If your thyroid levels are not normal, it is prudent to correct them before starting any other hormone balancing. Simply correcting a thyroid imbalance may improve your testosterone levels.

Supplementation can be started if the results show low levels of testosterone, progesterone, or DHEA, and especially if estradiol or DHT levels are on the high side. According to Dr. John Lee, the ratio of progesterone to estradiol in saliva in healthy young men is usually more than 200:1, and the testosterone to estradiol ratio is about 200 to 300:1. Pay particular attention to your ratios. Hormone levels tend to depend on each other, and the body will typically convert some hormones to others to maintain balance. Your supplementation plan should attempt to restore individual hormone levels to the correct range while keeping all hormone levels in their normal range.

Hormone Packaging

Hormones available for supplementation are often packaged as tablets, capsules, or creams. It is generally best to absorb hormones through the skin using a cream. Hormones passing through the digestive system (as capsules or tablets) have to be metabolized by the liver before they are available to the body. Higher doses are needed, and the liver has to break them down before the body can use them. Transdermal creams do not have this problem. According to Dr. Lee, it takes about seventy times as much oral hormone to reach the same concentration in the blood as absorbing it through the skin.[4] Thus, lower doses can be used, and they are absorbed quickly into the bloodstream. Many hormones are available for delivery this way, including progesterone, testosterone, and DHEA.

Lowering Estrogen Levels

Reducing estrogen levels is not always possible or practical. There are many herbs and foods that contain plant chemicals (phytoestrogens) that mimic human estrogen with less deleterious effects. Such herbal phytoestrogens can attach to estrogen receptors blocking some of the negative effects of estrogen. Several sources recommend the use of herbs like damiana (turnera aphrodisiaca or turnera diffusa) for this purpose, but while this herb has many valuable medicinal uses—particularly for women entering menopause—my personal belief is that it is of little value for male prostate dysfunction. In a man, aging does not alter estrogen levels significantly. The consensus of researchers is that aging causes a slight increase in estrogen level. In aging men significant increases in estrogen are more likely due to environmental or lifestyle issues. In Chapter Four I discussed ways to reduce the effects of environmental estrogens (xenoestrogens) on the body, along with lifestyle changes that will also help.

Blocking Effects of the Estrogens with Progesterone

Progesterone and testosterone are both often attracted to the same receptors on the prostate as estrogen. When either of them docks in an estrogen receptor, it effectively prevents the receptor from issuing estrogenic signals to the prostate. By restoring progesterone or testosterone levels—both of which tend to fall as a man ages—some of the negative effects of the estrogens can be blocked.[5, 6, 7]

As I mentioned in Chapter Three, estrogen, unopposed by progesterone or testosterone, is known to be a key player in the incidence of prostate and breast disease. Blocking some of its effects may cause a reversal of some prostate conditions—providing they are not too advanced. A study done in 1981 found that premenopausal women with low progesterone levels had more than a fivefold increase in risk of breast cancer and a tenfold increase in deaths from all cancers. This and other studies strongly suggest that progesterone deficiency is linked to various cancers.[8] Many of the studies referenced here suggest that testosterone deficiency has a similar effect.

It is easy to supplement with progesterone. In older men, a return to youthful progesterone levels can usually be achieved by a 6-8 mg per day application of a transdermal cream. This is about 1/16 to 1/8 of a teaspoon of cream containing 500 mg of progesterone per ounce. Since progesterone is a precursor to several hormones—one of which is testosterone—it can sometimes resolve symptoms by itself. Dr. Lee's recommendation is to try progesterone first and see if it helps. You can tell if it is working by how you feel. After a month or two, check your levels with a salivary hormone test and make adjustments if needed to keep your progesterone level in the normal range.

It is important to make sure that only natural or USP progesterone is used. Natural progesterone cream can be obtained over the counter from most health food stores, typically in two or four ounce jars or pump-top containers.

Dehydroepiandrosterone (DHEA) Supplementation

As we learned in Chapter Three, dehydroepiandrosterone (DHEA)—like progesterone—is a precursor to several other steroid hormones. It is found in almost all body tissues and is the most abundant hormone in the body. Low DHEA levels often coexist with low testosterone levels, but supplementation with DHEA does not usually increase testosterone levels. Like testosterone, DHEA has many roles in the human body though not all of them are understood. There is evidence that DHEA may help reduce depression, increase nerve communications, and help promote wound healing.

The role that a low DHEA level plays in inducing ED is not completely known. DHEA production tends to peak in adults between the ages of thirty and forty years, and begins a gradual decline at about 2 percent per year thereafter.[9] In a recent study, oral DHEA supplementation at a level of 50 mg per day produced a statistically significant improvement in erectile function in two of the four groups of men tested. Men who improved had either no organic erectile impairment or had high blood pressure. No improvement was seen in the groups with diabetes or neurological disorders.[10] Erectile dysfunction is related to the health of endothelial tissue that lines blood vessels. (See Chapter Nine.) DHEA supplementation appears to increase the health and viability of these tissues.[11, 12, 13]

In another randomized, double blind, placebo-controlled study by the same authors, forty healthy men with erectile dysfunction and low DHEA levels were tested. The group was split into two groups of twenty. One group was treated with 50 mg per day of

DHEA for six months and the other received a placebo. The treated group had a significant improvement in all categories of the International Index of Erectile Function (IIEF), which, at the time of the study, was a 15-item erectile function questionnaire.* Interestingly, DHEA treatment at this level did not appear to have any impact on testosterone levels or other factors that would negatively affect the prostate.[14, 15] This was also true in another study that used 100 mg per day for a six-month period.[16]

The Massachusetts Male Aging Study (MMAS), published in 1994, found DHEA to be the only hormone out of seventeen measured where low levels were consistently associated with erectile dysfunction.[17] In a study specifically designed to measure the effects of DHEA supplementation on older adults, supplementation at the fifty mg/day level had no significant effect on other steroid hormone levels, but restored DHEA to young adult values. Supplementation also had no significant effect on levels of luteinizing hormone, follicle-stimulating hormone, or thyroid hormones. A high percentage of the study participants reported an increased sense of well-being and improvements in libido and sexual ability. Other (nonsexual) effects of restoring DHEA to youthful levels were slight increases in bone density, skin hydration, and skin thickness.[18] Interestingly, several animal studies have found that DHEA offers protection against prostate cancer progression.[19] However, in these studies large amounts of DHEA (1000 to 2000 mg) were used, and while the results are interesting, there is no evidence that humans might have a similar response.

The effects of DHEA on the body appear to be independent of androgen levels. There is growing evidence that DHEA plays a significant role in increasing the availability of nitric oxide, and may also inhibit excess proliferation of smooth muscle cells, a process that has been implicated in the development of atherosclerosis.[20, 21] As we discussed earlier, low nitric oxide levels exacerbate existing ED, and atherosclerosis is strongly implicated in its

---

* The IIEF test has since been simplified to the standard IIEF-5 test shown in Chapter Nine.

development. DHEA also appears to reduce insulin resistance, thus it may help reduce abdominal obesity.[22, 23]

Like other hormones, you should only supplement with DHEA if your levels are low. If you are using it to help with erectile dysfunction, start with 25 mg per day. If after one month, you do not notice any appreciable increase in erectile performance, increase the daily dosage to 50 mg. If you are older than sixty, you may want to try taking up to 100 mg. However, as with many hormone supplements, it is wise to consult with your doctor about this. It is very unwise to exceed 100 mg per day of DHEA. If you have access to DHEA skin cream, by all means use it instead of capsules or tablets, but follow the accompanying instructions carefully. Much lower doses are typically needed with transdermal creams (see "Using Natural Hormones" in this chapter).

The Myth of Androstenedione

Androstenedione or "andro" is an over-the-counter product that has a bad reputation due to its misuse by many athletes and body builders. It is produced in the body from DHEA and is a direct precursor to both estrogen and testosterone. It can raise testosterone levels, and conversely, it can also raise estrogen levels. Excessive supplementation with andro can result in dangerous levels of both hormones and produce serious negative effects on the body, including excessive facial hair, acne, abnormal increases in male breast size (gynecomastia), testicular atrophy (shrinking testicles), priapism (painful unwanted erections), and possibly serious prostate problems. These and other problems have been noted with bodybuilders who have taken high doses of andro in an attempt to gain bulkier muscles.

There is no doubt that andro can temporarily raise testosterone levels. However, studies show that the percentage of testosterone increase caused by supplementation with andro is smaller than that of estradiol.[24] Secondly, since the testosterone increase occurs rapidly, the body senses this and turns off internal testosterone production. This is exactly opposite of the desired effect.

While the increased testosterone level might be temporarily helpful to correct ED problems, the eventual crash in testosterone production and the deleterious effects of increased estrogen can quickly negate any perceived gains.

Many websites and supplement manufacturers, particularly those aimed at building muscle mass, make much of the claim that supplemental androstenedione will significantly increase testosterone levels. Unfortunately, few of them provide any serious discussion of side effects or consequences. In one report, a man using andro for muscle building experienced an episode of priapism that lasted more than thirty hours and required medical treatment at a local emergency room.[25] The man had previously experienced a shorter bout of priapism that resolved spontaneously. He had no other risk factor for this condition.

In addition, quality double-blind studies have reported that there is little truth to the claim that supplementing with andro increases adaptation to resistance training.[26] And some studies have raised the possibility of liver damage as well as permanent disruption of the testosterone producing cells in the testicles with excessive androstenedione supplementation. Make no mistake, prolonged use of androstenedione, especially in high doses, can result in serious health issues, many of which are not reversible. There are far better—and safer—ways to balance your testosterone levels.

Bio-Identical Testosterone Supplementation

Testosterone is an extremely important hormone for the overall health of the human body and is particularly critical for male sexual ability and satisfaction. A recent large study noted an increase in general overall mortality of about 15 percent for men with low testosterone levels as compared to men with normal levels.[27]

Menopausal women can look to hundreds of plants and foods containing phytoestrogens that help to overcome age-related effects of dropping estrogen levels. Unfortunately, men do not have as large a selection. There are few herbs that can boost testosterone levels. In Chapter Nine, we mentioned three that are reputed to increase testosterone levels—ginseng, tribulus, and tongkat ali. Of the three, only ginseng has been extensively studied in humans, and it is the only herb that has a *proven* effect on testosterone levels. But the folklore on the others is quite strong, and there is some clinical evidence from animal studies. Keep in mind that, unless you have extremely low testosterone levels, natural techniques are more healthful than prescription testosterone shots or creams.

Testosterone is available only by prescription. Unlike progesterone, you cannot buy natural testosterone at your local health food store. Making it available over the counter would likely induce significant abuse among those who would attempt using it to enhance physical performance.

Many medical professionals frown on testosterone supplementation in any form. But the latest research suggests that this paradigm is wrong, and that low testosterone levels, particularly low free testosterone levels, are actually associated with prostate dysfunction. Recent studies have challenged the prevailing theory that testosterone supplementation in men with low levels of the hormone can initiate growth of a prostate tumor.[28, 29, 30, 31, 32, 33, 34]

Testosterone supplementation should only be done if one's levels are low, and you are having symptoms associated with low testosterone. In a study summary presented at the 2006 Annual Meeting of the American Urological Association, forty-one men were divided into two groups—one on testosterone therapy and the other on a placebo. At the end of the study, two men out of twenty-one in the testosterone group had developed prostate cancer, compared to four out of twenty in the placebo group. This small study is not enough to draw any specific conclusion regarding the risk of developing cancer, but there did not appear to be any detrimental effects of testosterone supplementation after six months. The study also noted that prostate levels of both DHT and testosterone increased in the blood, but similar increases did not occur in prostate tissue.[35]

While there is no evidence that testosterone replacement therapy can initiate prostate cancer, some researchers believe there is a theoretically increased risk. Since this is controversial, it is prudent that supplementation with testosterone be done only under the auspices of a medical professional who is up to date on such supplementation and after a thorough prostate exam to rule out cancer.

Testosterone deficiency contributes to low libido, reduced muscle mass, reduced bone mass, erectile dysfunction, atherosclerosis, and depression.[36, 37, 38] It is important to note that we are discussing free testosterone here and not total testosterone. Aging men often have low free testosterone levels with total testosterone levels in the normal range. Recent research has linked low free testosterone levels to the development of Alzheimer's disease, anemia, and an increased risk of diabetes.[39, 40, 41]

A common symptom of a low free testosterone level is an inability (or reduced ability) to have an orgasm during normal intercourse. Medically, this is known as anorgasmia or orgasmic dysfunction. While it can also be due to nerve desensitization, particularly

A note on injected testosterone

Testosterone introduced into the body via injection can cause some serious side effects. Typically, testosterone shots are given every two weeks to men with extremely low testosterone levels. The injection raises testosterone levels far beyond the normal biological ranges almost immediately. This causes the body to completely shut down testosterone production. The extremely high level slowly degrades as the body converts excess testosterone into other hormones like DHT and estrogen. For a few days an extremely high testosterone level occurs causing overstimulation by testosterone and higher levels of more dangerous hormones. It is my opinion that injected testosterone does more harm than good! The dosage of transdermal testosterone is more controllable and less harmful although it can still result in significant extremes in overall hormone balance. Unless your levels are extremely low, natural products offer the best alternative.

for diabetics, in most healthy men it is due to low free testosterone levels. Another common symptom is a lack of spontaneous erections during the night or early morning, which, barring other medical conditions, is almost always due to low free testosterone levels.

There appears to be two distinct chemical paths to spontaneous erections. The first is highly dependent on testosterone and the second dependent on nerve communication and other chemical signaling. Men with low free testosterone levels generally have missing or significantly less powerful nocturnal erections than men with normal levels. However, testosterone levels do not appear to directly effect erections induced by other erotic stimuli.[42, 43] Thus, while testosterone level is extremely important, it is but one player in this complex orchestra. If you are having sexual difficulties, and you are not experiencing spontaneous nocturnal or early morning erections, have both your total and free testosterone levels checked.

Adequate testosterone levels are essential for a man to have normal libido, orgasms, and spontaneous erections. Unfortunately, there is no specific value to determine what an adequate or normal level is. What is normal for one man may be woefully insufficient for another. If your testosterone levels fall on the low side of the normal range and you are having symptoms of low testosterone, replacement therapy may be in order, particularly if you are not experiencing nocturnal erections.

If you do have very low levels, it is advisable to see your doctor before doing anything natural. Low testosterone levels can be caused by a benign pituitary tumor or other conditions, and it is wise to rule these out first. If your levels are very low, and all medical causes are ruled out, your doctor can prescribe a bio-identical transdermal testosterone cream for you.

There are many different types of prescription testosterone therapies. The only one that is recommended is natural USP bio-identical testosterone cream.* This is typically available from a compounding pharmacy that prepares a concentration according to

---

* USP is an acronym for United States Pharmaceutical and indicates a pharmaceutical grade product.

your doctor's prescription. Other forms of testosterone, including intravenous shots and skin patches are often made of synthetic chemicals similar but not identical to natural testosterone. These are not fully recognized by the body and can have serious side effects, which include the possibility of liver damage. Biweekly intravenous injection of synthetic testosterone also raises testosterone levels far too high in the first few days after the injection and allows it to drop too low by the second week. This is nowhere near the normal function of the body and can cause significant problems.

The average man produces about 4 to 7 mg of testosterone per day in a circadian pattern.* Normal testosterone levels can usually be reached within a few weeks by using a low dose transdermal cream mixed by a compounding pharmacy to contain about 25 to 50 mg of testosterone per dose.[44] Typically, only about 10 percent of the dose is absorbed into the blood, so this will yield about 2.5 to 5 mg of testosterone per day. The International Academy of Compounding Pharmacists can help you locate both a doctor and a compounding pharmacy in your area. (See the appendix for more information.)

If you are using prescription testosterone cream, it is important to measure the dosage carefully. Testosterone is considerably stronger than progesterone and more is definitely not better. Concentrations may differ at different pharmacies, so the amount used must be carefully measured to deliver the desired dose. The goal is simply to bring your testosterone level back to normal. Remember, some testosterone is converted to DHT in the body, and it is also a precursor to estradiol. Increasing your testosterone level beyond a biological normal range could cause other problems, and a theoretically increased risk of prostate cancer. Supplementation to increase testosterone levels should only be done under the direction of your medical doctor and then only if you are having symptoms of low testosterone, and your levels are below or on the low side of normal.

---

* A circadian pattern (or circadian rhythm) is a biological process that repeats at 24-hour intervals.

According to the 27th edition of *Stedman's Medical Dictionary* the normal range for testosterone for a male is 280-1100 ng/dl. Generally accepted reference ranges for testosterone are usually grouped by age. These ranges often vary between laboratories, and there is a significant difference between the low value for an older man and the high value for a younger man. Typically, a normal level of free testosterone is between 1.5 to 2.9 percent of the total testosterone value. Consider supplementing if your free testosterone is on the low side and you are having symptoms of low testosterone, even if your total testosterone level is in the normal range. This is particularly true if you are older than sixty. Again, keep in mind that the reference values vary somewhat between laboratories. The determinant should be how you feel in conjunction with the laboratory values. Table 1 below shows the range of age-related values of total testosterone from a typical laboratory.

The interesting thing to note about these values is that the high limit of normal for a man over sixty is more than 30 percent below that of a thirty-nine year old. This brings us back to earlier discussions of what is normal and what is optimal. Some researchers consider that the values for young men are also valid for older men.[45, 46]

While you cannot buy high-dose testosterone cream without a prescription, you can find very low dose (homeopathic) creams available over the counter. Before you take the step to prescription testosterone replacement, you may want to try one of the over-the-counter products. They are generally inexpensive and often use a

TABLE 1 — Total Testosterone Range by Age

16 – 19 years	200 – 970 ng/dL
20 – 39 years	400 – 1080 ng/dL
40 – 59 years	350 – 890 ng/dL
Over 60 years	350 – 720 ng/dL

combination of herbal extracts along with homeopathic (very low dose) testosterone. For some men they can be effective at raising free testosterone without a corresponding increase in DHT or estradiol levels. I have listed one such cream on my website and will post others as they become available.

How to use Natural Hormones

The best way to supplement with hormones is to use bio-identical transdermal creams made specifically for that purpose. These creams typically use a liposome base that aids their absorption into the skin. When spread on thin-skinned areas of the body, they are quickly absorbed into the fatty parts of the skin tissue and transported into the blood stream. If you cannot find a transdermal cream for the particular hormone you want to use, seek a tablet form.

It is also important to rotate areas where the cream is used so that no particular skin area gets overused. Most hormones are stored in the fatty tissue layer just below the skin. If you continually use the same skin area day after day, the tissue can become saturated with the hormone and will absorb less of it. Aside from wasting the cream, it will result in less of the hormone getting into your bloodstream. The transdermal creams can be applied anywhere on the skin. Scrotal skin is particularly sensitive to progesterone and testosterone creams, but again, you should alternate sites.

Continuous supplementation with any hormone may cause the body to shut down internal production of that hormone. To prevent this, you should cycle hormone use. Typically, you use the hormone for about three weeks and then take a one-week break. The resulting deficit during the break triggers the body to turn up production of that hormone. Sometimes a few months of cycling may nudge the body to permanently increase production, thus eliminating the need for external supplementation. This is not proven, but I have heard cases of it happening, particularly with testosterone.

Tracking Your Response

When using supplemental hormones, it is essential to keep track of your body's response. Hormonal imbalances often occur many years before more evident symptoms of dysfunction appear, and it may take several months for your levels to come into balance. This is why it is important to measure your hormone levels prior to implementing a program to rebalance them. Establishing a record allows you to monitor and adjust your progress to best enhance your overall health. Excessive supplementation can cause serious problems, and insufficient supplementation will not be effective. The best way to track hormone levels is to test them before starting and repeat testing regularly at one or two month intervals. It is best to pick a laboratory for your testing and stick with it. Laboratories may have different equipment or testing protocols that may make results slightly different.

Saliva testing usually ranges in price from about $30 to $50 per hormone tested, so a typical test run for five hormones can average about two hundred dollars. However, unless your levels are badly out of range—which necessitates more frequent testing—it is usually adequate to test only once every six months. As you get better at regulating your supplementation plan, an annual test should be enough. You can also cut your long-term costs by dropping some hormones from the scheduled tests once you know they are staying in the correct range.

Summary

Hormone supplementation is not for everyone. If you do choose this method of rebalancing your hormones, it is essential to work closely with a qualified health professional who has experience in this area. Getting your hormones back in balance can be very rewarding. Remember that hormones are very powerful, and a little goes a long way. Also, remember that more is definitely not better, and excessive supplementation with hormones can be seriously damaging to your health.

Chapter Eleven

Putting it All Together

When I first began the quest to learn more about my prostate, I thought I would find a few specific items or lifestyle issues that would increase the likelihood of developing prostate disease. But as my knowledge grew, I realized that there are no specific items that cause such problems. As I have mentioned throughout this book, prostate disease, including cancer, results from multiple sources. Some of these are nutritional deficiencies (and excesses) and others are due to environmental issues, including chemical pollutants, stress, and aging. A multitude of studies have found various items with positive links to the development of prostate disorders, as well as a plethora of items that can protect one's prostate health. There is no evidence, however, that any single item either causes or protects one from developing prostate disease. It is my belief that the best approach to preventing or correcting prostate dysfunction naturally should address as many of the known causative—and preventative—factors as possible. In other words, if the cause is multifactorial—so should be the solution.

General Lifestyle Issues — Review

Men with prostate cancer are advised about treatment options but rarely advised to change their lifestyle and diet. It is generally agreed that the majority of prostate problems, including prostate cancer, could be prevented by dietary and lifestyle changes.[1, 2, 3]

Such changes also favor recovery from early, nonaggressive, prostate cancer as well. Unfortunately, some medical practitioners take an aggressive treatment approach even if their patient's cancer is of a grade unlikely to cause serious problems. This aggressive approach can cause a loss of quality of life for the patient far beyond that which might have resulted from a low-grade cancer. In a recent study, ninety-three men with early biopsy-proven prostate cancer who chose not to have any further medical treatment were randomly assigned to two groups. The first group (experimental group) was asked to make comprehensive changes in lifestyle and diet, while the second (control group) was not. After one year, none of the patients in the experimental group had to have additional treatment, while six patients in the control group had to undergo additional treatment due to progression of their disease. In addition, the experimental group had a decrease in PSA of 6 percent, while the control group had an average increase of 4 percent.[4]

Diet — Consuming a high animal fat, low vegetable, low fruit diet is associated with an increased risk for chronic illness, including prostate disease. A diet that is low in animal fat and abundant in fresh fruit and vegetables, nuts, seeds, and legumes, is associated with a decreased risk. Phytoestrogens in plants can help block the deleterious effects of estrogens produced by the body or absorbed through the environment. Also, a diet rich in plant foods can help substantially to balance hormone levels and reduce the risk of disease. Losing weight can also help you regain erectile function, especially if you are significantly overweight.[5]

A high intake of meat and dairy products in particular has been associated with a higher risk of developing prostate disease.[6, 7] Well-cooked meat, especially when cooked on a barbeque, has been linked to increased development of prostate cancer.[8, 9]

To reduce your risk of prostate problems you should decrease the amount of animal fat in your diet and increase your consumption of fruits, vegetables and plant fats, particularly those from nuts and seeds. Lycopene from cooked tomatoes in the form of sauces and purees is also protective. The fiber contained in vegetables is the most protective. One recent study found that men who consumed the highest overall amount of vegetable fiber had a significantly lower risk of prostate cancer than men who consumed the lowest.[10]

Reducing Xenoestrogens — To reduce the absorption and risk from xenoestrogens, minimize the use of plastic utensils, especially plastic wraps and soft plastic containers. Most plastic wraps are notorious for leeching xenoestrogens into foods wrapped in them. This is especially true for high-fat foods like cheese. Also, never heat or microwave foods in plastic containers or with plastic wrapped around them. Such practices inevitably drive xenoestrogens into the food, which are subsequently absorbed by your body. Minimize or eliminate the use of pesticides around your home and in your garden. Learn organic, pesticide-free gardening techniques. Home lawns and gardens can be maintained quite nicely without pesticides by using natural techniques to control pests. Certain plants, like marigolds, have a natural ability to repel pests, and are also aesthetically pleasing.

Stop Smoking — It is well-known that smoking contributes significantly to poor health. What many men who smoke do not realize is that smoking is also a significant risk factor for erectile dysfunction as well as many types of cancers. While many studies have not found an increased risk for prostate cancer or other prostate problems due to smoking, there is no question that smoking causes significant problems with sexual functioning.[11, 12]

Miscellaneous Items — Some medications are known to cause prostate problems. Antihistamines typically used in cold medicines can irritate the prostate, particularly if you suffer from prostatitis. Nonsteroidal anti-inflammatory drugs (NSAIDs) like ibuprofen, naproxin, and ketoprofen, found in over-the-counter products like Aleve, as well as prescription medications like Celebrex, can exacerbate urinary retention. According to a recent study, the risk of acute urinary retention is doubled in men who use NSAIDs.[13]* Any man with BPH and its corresponding urinary restrictions would be

---

* Acute urinary retention is a sudden inability to urinate. It can be quite painful and usually results in a visit to the emergency room for catheterization.

wise to avoid NSAIDs and antihistamines. If you are in doubt about a particular product, consult your doctor or your pharmacist.

Exercise, Fitness, and Immunity

Anything that stimulates the immune system can help your body prevent or reverse disease. It is well-known and conclusively proven that regular exercise builds a healthy immune system. Interestingly, prostate disease has been maintained by some researchers to be unassociated—or inconsistently associated—with levels of exercise. I do not subscribe to that belief. Since exercise is known to help build a healthy body, it is more than reasonable to conclude that exercise lowers the risk of all disease, including that of the prostate.

Some recent studies that examined prostate disease relative to physical activity on the job found that long-term sedentary employment increased risks, while employment requiring high levels of physical activity had a beneficial effect.[14, 15, 16, 17, 18] In addition, exercise has been shown to improve hormone balance and is certainly proven to enhance sexual function.[19, 20] While midlife changes in diet are beneficial, regular physical activity, even when initiated late in life, has the most significant effect towards reversing erectile dysfunction.[21]

It is wise to have a complete medical checkup before beginning a new exercise program, especially if you have a reputation for being a long-term couch potato. Exercise can temporarily increase PSA levels.[22] Thus, you should avoid strenuous exercise for at least twenty-four hours before having blood drawn for a diagnostic PSA test.

Drinking Water — The availability of clean drinking and cooking water and its relationship to disease cannot be understated. In many areas of the world, a lack of pure, clean water is a major cause of disease, primarily through water-borne bacteria. In the United States, waterborne bacteria are not as serious a problem due to extensive water purification. However, water is an excellent solvent, and many environmental pollutants are water-soluble. We need water to survive, but anything dissolved in it becomes part of us with each sip! Other toxins, such as many petrochemicals, are fat-soluble and enter our bodies through the foods we eat. And some, like asbestos fibers and auto exhaust, sneak in with the air we breathe. Many disease conditions can be attributed to an accumulation of toxins in the body. Regardless of how toxins enter the body, they can damage or destroy body organs and tissue if they accumulate in sufficient quantity.

Volatile industrial chemicals can also appear in our water supply. It is a good preventive measure to make sure your drinking and cooking water supply is as pure as possible. In my experience the best way to do this is to purchase a reverse-osmosis water purifier. Such units are inexpensive and can remove nearly all the dissolved solids from your water source. In addition, their carbon pre- and post-filters also remove the chlorine used by municipalities for sterilization.

Stress Reduction — It is well-known that stress is a major cause of illness, including, but not limited to, prostate disease. Stress can come from many sources. We usually relate stress to emotional conditions, but in reality it is anything that disturbs the normal function of the body. A good example of this occurs in people who work rotating shifts. The body is continually stressed due to the absence of a stable daily schedule. A recent large-scale study of 14,052 men in Japan found that rotating shift workers had a significantly increased risk of developing prostate cancer of about three to one. Men who worked continuous night shifts had a small, but insignificant increase in risk.[23]

Environmental toxins stress the body in a different way by making the organs of elimination work harder, and emotional stress has a direct effect on hormone levels. Regardless of the source, all stress takes energy away from other important processes like healing, and has a major effect on hormone balance. It causes cortisol levels to rise and other hormones to drop. When stress is temporary, as with a sudden fright or physical exercise, hormone levels return to normal relatively quickly. However, continuous unrelenting stress keeps our hormones in a perpetual unbalanced state and can lead to serious illness. To avoid this, it is imperative to make lifestyle changes that will reduce stress as much as possible.

Stimulating Immunity — Improving immunity is another powerful technique in the prevention of disease. Improving your diet to one that consists mostly of vegetables and fruits is a good starting point. There are also many herbs of proven value that will stimulate and improve immunity on a long-term basis. Many of the techniques discussed in the previous chapters for balancing hormones will also help improve immunity. Remember, hormonal imbalance comes from many sources, including stress and environmental toxins. When your hormones are imbalanced, immunity is compromised. And an immune system that is not functioning at a peak level provides an environment for disease to flourish. Frequent illness increases stress on the body—and more stress precipitates further deterioration of immunity—a vicious cycle! Environmental toxins can have the same effect. Simply reducing stress and environmental toxin loading can help correct many problems and improve your overall health.

Selecting a Multivitamin

Throughout this book, I have provided detailed information on specific vitamins, minerals, and herbs that have been shown, either by clinical studies or extensive folklore, to be valuable for prostate health. Of course, one need only glance at the crowded shelves of any health food store to know there are many other supplements available. While some of these are of significant value, many have little to recommend them other than the claims of the manufacturer.

Table 1 on the next page shows some of the common vitamins and minerals that you should take to maintain or improve your general health along with their recommended daily levels. Most can be found in a high quality multivitamin product, although the quantities may vary. Note that this table shows supplements suggested for general health as well as some supplements—like selenium,

TABLE 1 — Common Vitamins and Minerals

Description	Daily Value
Vitamin A as beta-carotene	5000-10,000 IU
Vitamin A as retinyl palmitate	5000 IU max.
Vitamin B Complex (see note 1 below)	50 mg
Vitamin C	1000 mg
Vitamin D as (see Chapter 5)	800 IU
Vitamin E (see Chapter 6 and note 5)	800 IU
Vitamin K (See note 4)	200 mcg
Boron	500 mcg
Calcium as calcium citrate	1200 mg
Choline (see note 2 below)	100 mg
Chromium	100 mcg
Copper	1 mg
Inositol (see note 2 below)	50 mg
Iron (see note 3 below)	4 to 8 mg
Iodine	150 mcg
Magnesium as magnesium citrate	600 mg
Manganese	4 mg
Molybdenum	50 mcg
PABA (para-aminobenzoic acid) (see note 2 below)	50mg
Potassium	50 mg
Selenium (see Chapter 7)	200 mcg
Silicone	4 mg
Zinc (see Chapter 7)	50 mg

Note 1 — Vitamin B consists of a group of several similar vitamins. When first discovered, it was considered a single vitamin and thus named vitamin B. It has since been shown to be a family of related vitamins that typically appear together in various foods. To date, about twenty-two B vitamins have been isolated. Most multivitamins contain the important B vitamins in small amounts. These are thiamin (B_1) riboflavin (B_2) niacin (B_3) panthothenic acid (B_5) pyridoxine (B_6) biotin (B_7) folic acid (B_9) and cyanocobalamin (B_{12}). Most "B-Complex" products and some multivitamins provide 100% or more of the daily requirement of all needed B vitamins. This vitamin group is water-soluble. Doses that exceed the body's needs are eliminated in the urine—typically resulting in urine that is a bright yellow color.

Note 2 — Choline, inositol, and PABA are usually components of most B-complex products and are sometimes included in multivitamin products.

Note 3 — Too much or too little iron can cause problems. It is best to get most of your iron from food. Plant sources of iron are not absorbed as well as animal sources. The RDA for iron is 18 mg for adults, but that is probably higher than most people need.

Note 4 — Vitamin K can interfere with blood thinning medications. If you are on any kind of blood thinner, check with your doctor before using a multi containing vitamin K.

Note 5 — Most multivitamins contain 200 to 400 IU of vitamin E as D-alpha-tocopherol. For general prostate health, add a separate vitamin E supplement that contains all eight vitamin E fractions in natural form. (See Chapter Six).

zinc, and vitamin E—that are specific for prostate health and were discussed in detail earlier in this book. The idea is to take a high quality multivitamin and add other vitamins, minerals, or herbs to create a nutrient package that is customized for your specific needs. You will also note that there are significant differences between the daily values in Table 1 and the recommended daily allowances (RDAs) that you may find elsewhere. The recommended values in Table 1 are the results of my personal research and experience. In most cases, they are considerably higher then the usual RDAs discussed back in Chapter Three. A notable exception is potassium with an RDA of about five grams (5000 mg) for which table shows a value of 50 mg. Potassium is best obtained from eating fruits and vegetables, which have universally high potassium content. More specific nutrient information can be found in several websites listed in the appendix and some books in the bibliography.

While there are no specific vitamin deficiencies that have been linked to prostate problems, some deficiencies have been linked to the development of more aggressive disease. A deficiency of one of the B-vitamins, namely folate (B_9) has been linked to the development of aggressive prostate cancer.[24] There is also some evidence that older adults may need significantly more than the RDA of certain B-vitamins.[25] This is particularly true of Vitamin B_{12}. Excess amounts of B-vitamins are excreted in the urine. A little extra is not harmful.

Many multivitamins add various other minerals, digestive enzymes, and herbal items. Often, there is no evidence that they are needed, and the typical low quantities in a multivitamin are of little value even for those that are useful. There are also several terms supplement manufacturers use to help sell their products. Typically, they are called: high potency, energy, performance, senior or stress formulas. Ignore this advertising hype. Select a multivitamin from a reputable manufacturer that comes closest to supplying the values for the items shown in Table One.

Since it is impossible to pack all needed nutrients into a single pill, many of the better multivitamins list two to six tablets for one serving. Read the labels carefully. You may need to take several tablets to reach the desired amounts. If the product you select does not have the recommended amount of a specific nutrient, you can add that nutrient separately. This typically occurs with calcium and magnesium, and sometimes also with selenium and zinc. Calcium and magnesium are bulky, and some supplement manufacturers tend to use low values so that you can take fewer pills. For proper balance, the ratio of calcium to magnesium should always be about two to one.

Keep in mind that it is always best to get the bulk of your vitamin and mineral needs from foods. There are many good books available that can help you create a healthy diet for yourself. Several are listed in the bibliography.

Creating a Supplement Plan and Monitoring Your Progress

Once you have selected a multivitamin and mineral product for the common nutrients as described above, you can add other supplements that are beneficial for your specific needs. If you are trying to improve a specific prostate problem, refer to Chapters Six through Ten and decide which herbals are most likely to help you. It is best that you add only one or two items at a time to your supplement plan, particularly if the items have similar effects.

Many herbs and nutrients do their work slowly, often over a period of several months, so it is essential to keep track of your progress. This is especially true for herbs used to help with BPH, prostatitis, or to improve urinary flow. The easiest way to do this is to keep a log of any changes you make to your supplement plan as well as any changes you note in your symptoms. A good rule of thumb is to wait thirty to sixty days between significant changes.

One way to track your progress, particularly if you have been diagnosed with BPH, is to track any changes in your prostate symptoms using the International Prostate Symptom Score (IPSS) test shown in Table Two on the next page.[26]

TABLE 2 — International Prostate Symptom Score

Question	Score
During the last month or so, how often have you had a sensation of not emptying your bladder completely after you finish urinating?	
During the last month or so, how often have you had to urinate again less than two hours after you finished urinating?	
During the last month or so, how often have you found you stopped and started again several times when you urinated?	
During the last month or so, how difficult have you found it to postpone urination?	
During the last month or so, how often have you had a weak urinary stream?	
During the last month or so, how often have you had to push, strain, or wait to begin urination?	
During the last month or so, how many times did you typically get up to urinate from the time you went to bed until you got up in the morning?	
	Total =

To get your score, answer the first six questions on a scale of zero to five as follows:

0 = Not at all
1 = Less than 1 time in 5
2 = Less than half the time
3 = About half the time
4 = More than half the time
5 = Almost always.

Answer the last question with the actual times you woke to urinate. A score of zero to seven indicates mild dysfunction, eight to nineteen is moderate dysfunction, and above twenty is severe dysfunction.

Take the test and record your score before you start your supplement plan, and then every thirty days thereafter. When I first started supplementing for my prostate problems several years ago, my IPSS score was around twenty-seven. Currently, it runs about nine.

Always remember that there is no level of vitamin, mineral, or herbal supplementation that can overcome the negative effects of a poor diet! If you want to recover your health, it is essential that you change your lifestyle and eating habits. Dietary supplements should be viewed only as enhancements to a good diet.

Avoiding Common Pitfalls

Watch out for supplements that claim unusual benefits. Keep in mind the old adage, *"If it sounds too good to be true—it probably is."* Many manufacturers make claims for their products that have little resemblance to the truth. Watch the Daily Value (DV) recommendations for all supplements. Often the daily value is woefully inadequate, particularly if you are trying to solve a problem. As I mentioned in Chapter Seven, the recommended daily allowance (RDA) for some supplements is often not in sync with the latest research and is sometimes significantly lower than the optimal daily allowance (ODA). However, do not be lulled into thinking more is better. Many supplements can be harmful when taken in higher than recommended quantities. The best way to keep from taking too much or too little is to take the advice of experts and make sure that advice is current. There is much research being done on nutrients, and the values of a few years ago may be obsolete today. Check the websites listed in the appendix for the latest information on optimal daily nutrient requirements.

Conclusion

There are areas in this book where I have taken a position that may be contrary to the opinion of some medical practitioners. These opinions are mine and were derived from clinical and other reports I have read as well as my own experiences. My opinions are not meant to substitute for the advice of a licensed medical practitioner. They are for educational purposes only, and I strongly urge you to do your own research.

There is much controversy about the role that lack of sun exposure and low testosterone levels play in the development of prostate cancer. I believe that deficiencies in both are powerful risk factors, but there are others who disagree. It often takes many years for controversial ideas to gain acceptance, particularly in the medical profession. The conclusions and recommendations in this book are the result of my personal analysis of many, up-to-date, peer-reviewed, reports published in respected medical journals. However, I do admit that I am biased towards natural solutions.

The most significant difference between this book and conventional beliefs is in the area of testosterone supplementation. Conventional medicine is cautious regarding anything that might increase a man's androgen levels, such as direct replacement of testosterone, progesterone, DHEA, or any other testosterone precursor. In my opinion, when men with low androgen levels are given supplements, not only do their sex drives and abilities return to normal, but in many cases their overall health takes a major turn for the better. Several studies referenced in this book suggest that low free testosterone levels lead to prostate dysfunction—including prostate cancer. It is my belief that a significant drop in androgens—particularly testosterone—is one of the risk factors rather than one of the causes of prostate disease and many other chronic conditions. However, while prostate dysfunction is the focus of this book, it is very interesting to note that low levels of testosterone and other androgens are also associated with other chronic disorders. Convincing evidence for the latter comes from two recent studies. One looked at androgen deficiencies and chronic heart failure, and the other compared testosterone levels to physical performance and fall risk in older men. The first concluded that men suffering from chronic heart conditions are also deficient in total and free testosterone as well as other androgens, and that their overall prognosis was directly related to the amount of these deficiencies. The second found that older men with the lowest testosterone levels had reduced physical performance and fell more often, increasing their risk of injury substantially.[27, 28]

In 1941, Dr. Huggins proved that castration (surgical removal of the testicles) slowed progression of existing metastatic prostate cancer.[29]* This slowing was attributed to a significant decrease in testosterone levels due to the surgery. It is well-known that castration eliminates nearly all testosterone production, but it also causes significant alteration of many other hormones and the body processes that depend on them. Dr. Huggins findings—in a small study limited to men with prostate cancer that had already spread beyond the gland—have been extrapolated by some into the conclusion that testosterone causes prostate cancer. Recent studies I have examined dispute this, finding instead that low testosterone, particularly low free testosterone, is instead a risk factor for developing prostate cancer. Unfortunately, many professionals still believe testosterone is a causal agent.

In 1776, Thomas Paine wrote in "Common Sense:"

> A long habit of not thinking a thing wrong, gives it a superficial appearance of being right, and raises at first a formidable outcry in defense of custom. But the tumult soon subsides. Time makes more converts than reason.

Unfortunately, this long-held belief causes some professionals to overlook testosterone replacement therapy for cancer-free aging men with clear symptoms of hormone deficiency. In practice it is rarely considered as a preventative measure—even for men with normal prostates and no sign of prostate disease. And hormone

---

* The medical term for castration is orchiectomy.

balancing is rarely considered as part of a treatment plan *for* low-level prostate disease.

Many professions have high inertia when it comes to new ideas, even when the new ideas come from highly respected members of the community. In medicine this inertia can result in inadvertent harm to its patients. In the mid-19th century, Hungarian physician Ignaz Philipp Semmelweis was abused, criticized, and ostracized for his promotion of the idea that doctors should wash their hands after delivering an infant. He suggested that the death of many mothers due to fevers after childbirth was caused by the failure of physicians to wash their hands between deliveries. It was more than two decades before his ideas were even partially accepted—even though he significantly reduced the incidence of both mother and infant mortality by implementing this procedure in his clinics. Today, Semmilwies is considered to be one of the great physicians of his time. One can only wonder how many mothers and infants of that era suffered and died needlessly until his ideas were implemented. Unfortunately, cases like this abound with stunning frequency in medical history.

In the United States we are privileged to have the most sophisticated diagnostic equipment, but even with this technological advantage we lag far behind other countries in the incidence and treatment of chronic illnesses.[30] Much of this can be attributed to our lack of interest in natural healthy lifestyles and nutrition, our obsession with highly processed fast foods that have little nutritional value, and our belief, reinforced by daily pharmaceutical advertisements, that there is a pill for every illness.

Nearly 2,500 years ago, Hippocrates, "The Father of Medicine," offered this simple advice:

"Let food be thy medicine and let thy medicine be thy food."

Appendix

Websites for Additional Information

Many of the websites listed below are nonprofit organizations run by concerned citizens and doctors. I have limited the list to informative websites that are not overly technical.

Each of the websites listed here, and others added after this book was published, as well as the latest news about natural health and prostate problems, can be accessed instantly via the "Links" and "News" buttons on my website at http://www.ProstateHealth Naturally.com.

General Information on Vitamins, Minerals, Herbs, and Alternative Medicine

Alternative Medicine Foundation, Inc. — A nonprofit organization providing responsible, evidence-based information on the integration of alternative and conventional medicine. (See HerbMed) http://www.amfoundation.org

Consumer Laboratories — A subscription website that tests supplements for content and purity and provides this information to its subscribers. A substantial portion of the site is free. Claims to be the leading provider of independent test results and information to help consumers and healthcare professionals evaluate health, wellness, and nutrition products. http://www.consumerlab.com

Dr. Joseph Mercola's Website — A popular alternative medicine and natural health information site. Free newsletter available. Comprehensive medical and alternative health information. http://www.mercola.com

Healing Food Reference Database — A comprehensive resource with cross-referenced information about healing foods and the conditions they may help. http://www.healingfoodreference.com/

Healing Herbs Reference Database — Companion website for healing foods above. Provides cross-referenced information on herbs and conditions they may help. http://www.herbreference.com

HerbMed — An interactive, electronic herbal database that provides free hyperlinked access to the scientific data underlying the use of about forty popular herbs. The nonprofit Alternative Medicine Foundation, Inc. provides the site. An enhanced paid subscription site provides access to the entire database with continuous updating. http://www.herbmed.org

Linus Pauling Institute of Oregon State University. Micronutrient Information Center (MIC). The Institute functions from the basic premise that an optimum diet is the key to optimum health. The site provides detailed scientific information and recommendations on vitamins, minerals, and other nutrients, as well as a free research newsletter. http://lpi.oregonstate.edu/infocenter

MedLine — Information on virtually everything related to health. Maintained by the U.S. National Library of Medicine and the National Institutes of Health. http://medlineplus.gov

News Target — Provides news, interviews and product reviews on natural health, green living, and the environment. The site claims no financial relationships whatsoever with the nutritional products they write about or recommend, nor do they sell any such products. A free newsletter and many free reports are available. http://www.newstarget.com

SunlightD.org — An informational site about sunlight and Vitamin D from Krispin Sullivan, CN. http://sunlightandvitamind.com

Supplement Watch — A subscription website that tests supplements for content and purity and provides this information to its subscribers. A substantial portion of the site is free. http://www.supplementwatch.com

USDA National Nutrient Database — Provides search tools for finding nutrients or foods in the database by either content or name. http://www.nal.usda.gov/fnic/foodcomp/search/index.html

U.S. Department of Agriculture, Food and Nutrition Center — The Food and Nutrition Information Center (FNIC) website contains over 2000 links to current and reliable nutrition information. http://fnic.nal.usda.gov

Vitamin D Council — Run by a group of concerned citizens that believe many humans are needlessly suffering and dying from vitamin D deficiency. Site provides detailed information about Vitamin D requirements and supplementation as well as a free newsletter. http://www.vitamindcouncil.com

Prostate Cancer and Men's Health Topics

About Prostate Cancer — Subsite of the N.Y. Times "About.com" website. General site for prostate and other medical information. Publishes abstracts of latest reports on prostate cancer and other related conditions. http://prostatecancer.about.com

American Cancer Society. — General information on all types of cancer. http://www.cancer.org

American Foundation for Urologic Disease — General information about urology problems. Patient information and links to find a urologist. http://www.auafoundation.org

American Institute for Cancer Research (AICR) — A cancer charity that fosters research on diet and cancer prevention and educates the public about the results. http://www.aicr.org

Digital Urology Journal — An online journal with research articles on urologic problems. http://www.duj.com

National Association for Continence (NAFC) — Offers free literature about incontinence and referrals to physician specialists. http://www.nafc.org

National Cancer Institute — A government site for cancer information. http://www.nci.nih.gov

Prostate Cancer Research Institute — An organization for men with prostate cancer. Maintains a staffed help-line for free personal advice from experts. Free newsletter. http://prostate-cancer.org

Prostate Cancer Foundation (PCF) website — Formerly CaPCURE, the Prostate Cancer Foundation (PCF) is the world's largest philanthropic source of support for prostate cancer research. http://www.prostatecancerfoundation.org

PSA Rising — A site providing prostate cancer and nutrition news, information, and support. Has handy decision chart regarding risk associated with rising PSAs. http://www.psa-rising.com

Simon Foundation for Continence — A nonprofit organization dedicated to the topic of incontinence. http://www.simonfoundation.org

University of California, San Francisco — Comprehensive Cancer Center. Many free research articles on nutrition and cancer available for download in PDF format. http://cancer.ucsf.edu

Hormone Testing Laboratories and Pharmacies

AllVia Integrative Pharmaceuticals, Inc. — Performs salivary hormone testing. Also sells several transdermal hormone creams and other natural products. 11202 N. 24th Ave, Phoenix, AZ 85029, Phone 877-995-8715, Fax: 602-424-0464. http://www.allviahealth.com

Diagnos-Tech, Inc. — Performs salivary hormone testing. Also sells several transdermal hormone creams and other natural products. 6620 S. 192nd Place, Kent, WA 98032, 425-251-0596, 800-878-3787. http://www.diagnostechs.com/main.htm

International Academy of Compounding Pharmacists — Provides a list of compounding pharmacists who can refer you to local doctors that prescribe natural hormones. P.O. Box 1365, Sugar Land, TX 77487, Phone: 281-933-8400, Toll-Free Referral Line 800-927-4227 Fax: 281-495-0602. http://www.iacprx.org

ZRT Laboratory, LLC — Performs salivary hormone testing for the sex steroid hormones. Also sells several transdermal hormone creams. 1815 NW 169th Pl. # 5050, Beaverton, OR 97006, 503-466-2445. http://www.zrtlab.com/

References

Chapter 1

1 Shigemurs, K., et al. "Larger prostate causes higher frequency of infectious complications in prostate biopsy," *Urologia Internationalis*, Vol. 76, No. 4 (May 2006), 321-326.

Chapter 2

1 Balch, James F., Phyllis Balch, *Prescription for Nutritional Healing*, 3rd ed. (New York: Avery Books, 2000).

2 Feldman, H.A., et al. "Massachusetts Male Aging Study," *Journal of Urology*, Vol. 151, No. 1 (Jan 1994); 54-61.

3 Ming, W., et al., "Total Cholesterol and High Density Lipoprotein Cholesterol as Important Predictors of Erectile Dysfunction," *American Journal of Epidemiology*, Vol. 140, No. 10 (July 1994); 930-937,

4 Grover, S., et al. "The Prevalence of Erectile Dysfunction in the Primary Care Setting," *Archives of Internal Medicine*, Vol. 166, No. 2 (Jan. 2006); 213-219.

5 Pienta, K., et al, "Risk Factors for Prostate Cancer. *Annals of Internal Medicine*, Vol. 118, No. 10 (May 1993);793-803.

6 Gupta, S., et al. "Chronic Inflammation Linked With Start of Prostate Cancer: A 5 Year Follow Up Study," 97th Annual Meeting of the American Association for Cancer Research, (April 2006).

7 ———. "Chronic Inflammation of the Prostate and Development of Prostate Cancer," *Journal of Urology*, Vol. 176 (Oct. 2006);1012-1016.

8 Faigin, R., *Natural Hormone Enhancement* (Northborough, MA: Extique Publishing, 2000), p. 327.

9 Shippen, E., Fryer, W., *The Testosterone Syndrome* (New York: M. Evans and Company, 1998), p. 98.

Chapter 3

1 Stattin, P., et al. "High Levels of Circulating Testosterone are not Associated with Increased Prostate Cancer Risk: a Pooled Prospective Study, *International Journal of Cancer.* Vol. 108, No. 3 (Jan 2004); 418-424.

2 Raivio, T., et al, "Reduced Circulating Androgen Bioactivity in Patients with Prostate Cancer," *Prostate*, Vol. 55, No. 3 (May 2003); 194-198.

3 Wu, A., et al., "Serum Androgens and Sex Hormone-Binding Globulins in Relation to Lifestyle Factors in Older African-American, White and Asian Men in the United States and Canada," *Cancer Epidemiol Biomarkers Preview,* Vol. 4, No. 7 (Oct.-Nov. 1995); 735-741.

4 Imperato-McGinley, J, et al, "Prostate Visualization Studies in Males Homozygous and Heterozygous for 5-Alpha-Reductase Deficiency," *The Journal of Clinical Endocrinology and Metabolism,* Vol. 75, No. 4 (Oct. 1992); 1022-1026.

5 Hetts, S., "To Die or Not to Die: An Overview of Apoptosis and its Role in Disease," *Journal of the American Medical Association,* Vol. 279, No. 4 (Jan. 1998); 300-307.

6 Ross, R., et al. "Do Diet and Androgens Alter Prostate Cancer Risk via a Common Etiologic Pathway?" *Journal of the National Cancer Institute,* Vol. 86, No.4 (Feb. 1994); 252-254.

7 Castagnetta, L., et al, "Growth of LNCaP Human Prostate Cancer Cells is Stimulated by Estradiol Via Its Own Receptor," *Endocrinology,* Vol. 136, No. 5 (1995); 2309-2319.

8 Hess, R.A., et al, "A Role For Oestrogens in the Male Reproductive System," *Nature,* Vol. 390 (Dec. 1997); 509-512.

9 Harman, S.M., et al. "Longitudinal Effects of Aging on Serum Total and Free Testosterone Levels in Healthy Men," *The Journal of Clinical Endocrinology & Metabolism,* Vol. 86, No. 2 (Feb. 2001); 724-731.

10 Morley, J.E., et al. "Longitudinal Changes in Testosterone, Luteinizing Hormone, and Follicle-Stimulating Hormone in Healthy Older Men," *Metabolism: clinical and experimental,* Vol. 46, No. 4 (April 1997); 410-413.

11 Nakhla, A., et al. "Stimulation of Prostate Cancer Growth by Androgens and Estrogens Through the Intermediacy of Sex Hormone-Binding Globulin," *Endocrinology,* Vol. 137, No. 10 (Oct. 1996); 4126-4129.

12 Nakhla, A., et al. "Estradiol Causes the Rapid Accumulation of cAMP in Human Prostate," *Proceedings of the National Academy of Science, U S A.,*Vol. 91, No. 12 (June 1994); 5402-5405.

13 Farnsworth WE, "Roles of Estrogen and SHBG in Prostate Physiology, *Prostate,* Vol. 28, No. 1 (Jan. 1996); 17-23.

14 Yang N, et al, "Identification of an Estrogen Response Element Activated by Metabolites of 17B-Estradiol and Raloxifen. *Science,* Vol. 273, No. 5279 (Aug. 1996); 1222-1225.

15 Bonkhoff, H., et al. "Implications of Estrogens and Their Receptors for the Development and Progression of Prostate Cancer," *Der Pathologe,* Vol. 26, No. 6 (Nov. 2005); 461-468.

16 Stoff, J. *The Prostate Miracle*, (New York: Kensington Health, 2000), p. 214.

[17] Faigin, R. *Natural Hormone Enhancement* (Cedar Mountain, N.C., Extique Publishing, 2000), p 328.

[18] Formby, B., et al. "Progesterone Inhibits Growth and Induces Apoptosis in Breast Cancer Cells: Inverse Effects on Bcl-2 and p53," *Annals of Clinical & Laboratory Science,* Vol. 28, No. 6 (Nov.-Dec. 1998); 360-369.

[19] ———. Bcl-2, Surviving and Variant CD44 v7-v10 are Downregulated and p53 is Upregulated in Breast Cancer Cells by Progesterone: Inhibition of Cell Growth and Induction of Apoptosis," *Molecular and Cellular Biochemistry,* Vol. 202, No. 1-2 (Dec. 1999); 53-61.

[20] Lee, J. *Natural Progesterone: The Multiple Roles of a Remarkable Hormone,* (Charlbury, U.K., Jon Carpenter Publishing, 2002), 2nd Ed.

Chapter 4

[1] Sharpe, R., et al. "How Strong is the Evidence of a Link Between Environmental Chemicals and Adverse Effects on Human Reproductive Health?" *British Medical Journal,* Vol. 328 (Feb. 2004); 447-451.

[2] Lee, John, *Natural Progesterone, Multiple Roles of a Remarkable Hormone,* 2nd Ed, 1999 (Chalbury, UK: Jon Carpenter Publishing, Market Street, [date]), pp. 45, 48-49, 65, 93.

[3] *Discover Magazine,* August 2003, p. 16.

[4] Archibeque-Engle, S., et al. "Comparison of Organochlorine Pesticide and Polychlorinated Biphenyl Residues in Human Breast Adipose Tissue and Serum," *Journal of Toxicology and Environmental Health,* Vol. 52, No. 4 (Nov. 1997); 285-293.

[5] Armstrong, B., et al. "Environmental Factors and Cancer Incidence and Mortality in Different Countries, With Special References to Dietary Practices," *International Journal of Cancer,* Vol. 15, No. 4 (April 1975); 617-631.

[6] Rose, D., et al. "International Comparisons of Mortality Rates for Cancer of the Breast, Ovary, Prostate, and Colon, and Per Capita Food Consumption," *Cancer,* Vol. 58, No. 11 (Dec. 1986); 2363-2371.

[7] Lee, M., et al, "Case-Control Study of Diet and Prostate Cancer in China," *Cancer Causes Control,* Vol. 9. No. 6 (Dec. 1998); 545-552.

[8] Giovannucci, E., et al, "A Prospective Study of Dietary Fat and Risk of Prostate Cancer," *Journal of the National Cancer Institute,* Vol. 85, No. 19 (Oct. 1993); 1571-1579.

[9] Giovannucci, E., et al. "A Prospective Study of Calcium Intake and Incident and Fatal Prostate Cancer," *Cancer Epidemiology Biomarkers & Prevention,* Vol. 15 (Feb. 2006); 203-210.

[10] Gao, X., et al. "Prospective Studies of Dairy Product and Calcium Intakes and Prostate Cancer Risk: a Meta-Analysis," *Journal of the National Cancer Institute,* Vol. 97, No. 23 (Dec. 2005); 1768-1777.

11 Whitmore, A.S., et al. "Prostate Cancer in Relation to Diet, Physical Activity, and Body Size in Blacks, Whites, and Asians in the United States and Canada,"*Journal of the National Cancer Institute*, Vol. 87, No. 9 (May 1995); 654-661.

12 Freedland, S., et al. "Stronger Association Between Obesity and Biochemical Progression after Radical Prostatectomy Among Men Treated in the Last 10 Years," *Clinical Cancer Research*, Vol. 11 (April 2005); 2883-2888.

13 Kolonel, L., et al. "Vegetables, Fruits, Legumes and Prostate Cancer: A Multiethnic Case-Control Study," *Cancer Epidemiology Biomarkers & Prevention*, Vol. 9 (Aug. 2000); 795-804.

14 Chan, J., et al. "Role of Diet in Prostate Cancer Development and Progression," *Journal of Clinical Oncology*, Vol. 23, No. 32 (Nov. 2005); 8152-8160.

15 Kaul, L., et al. "The Role of Diet in Prostate Cancer, *Nutrition and Cancer,* Vol. 9, No. 2-3 (1987); 123-128.

16 Slattery, M.L., et al. "Food-Consumption Trends Between Adolescent and Adult Years and Subsequent Risk of Prostate Cancer," *The American Journal of Clinical Nutrition,* Vol. 52, No. 4 (Oct. 1990); 752-757.

17 Snowdon, D.A. "Diet, Obesity, and Risk of Fatal Prostate Cancer," *American Journal of Epidemiology,* Vol. 120, No. 2 (Aug. 1984); 244-250.

18 Freedland, S., et al. "Obesity and Risk of Biochemical Progression Following Radical Prostatectomy at a Tertiary Care Referral Center," *Journal of Urology,* Vol. 174, No. 3 (Sept. 2005); 919-922.

19 MacInnis, R.J., et al, "Body Size and Composition and Prostate Cancer Risk," *Cancer Epidemiology Biomarkers & Prevention,* Vol. 12 (Dec. 2003); 1417-1421.

20 Fletcher, R., et al. "Vitamins for Chronic Disease Prevention in Adults," *Journal of the American Medical Association,* Vol. 287, No. 23 (June 2002); 3127-3129.

21 Sesso, H., et al. "Alcohol Consumption and Risk of Prostate Cancer: The Harvard Alumni Health Study," *International Journal of Epidemiology,* Vol. 30 (2001); 749-755.

22 Hayes, R.B., et al. "Alcohol Use and Prostate Cancer Risk in US Blacks and Whites," *American Journal of Epidemiology,* Vol 143, No. 7 (Jan. 1996); 692-697.

23 Couwenbergs, C. J. "Acute Effects of Drinking Beer or Wine on the Steroid Hormones of Healthy Men," *Journal of Steroid Biochemistry,* Vol. 31, No. 4A (Oct. 1988); 467–467.

24 M. C. Bosland, "The Role of Steroid Hormones in Prostate Carcinogenesis, Chapter 2," *Journal of the National Cancer Institute: Monographs,* Vol. 2000, No. 27 (July 2000); 39-66.

25 Faigin, R, *Natural Hormone Enhancement,* (Cedar Mountain, N.C., Extique Publishing, 2000), p. 328.

26 Henderson, B. E., et al. "Endogenous Hormones as a Major Factor in Human Cancer," *Cancer Research,* Vol. 42 (Aug. 1982); 3232-3239.

27 Jeong-Youn, J., et al. "Effects of Grape Cell Culture Extracts on Human Topoisomerase II Catalytic Activity and Characterization of Active Fractions," *Journal of Agricultural and Food Chemistry,* Vol. 53, No. 7 (April 2005); 2489-2498.

28 Jang, M., et al. "Cancer Chemopreventive Activity of Resveratrol, a Natural Product Derived from Grapes," *Science Magazine,* Vol. 275, No. 5297 (Jan. 1997); 218 – 220.

29 Cerhan, J., et al. "Association of Smoking, Body Mass, and Physical Activity with Risk of Prostate Cancer in the Iowa 65+ Rural Health Study (United States)," *Cancer Causes Control,* Vol. 8, No. 2 (March 1997); 229-238.

30 Giovannucci, E., et al, "Smoking and Risk of Total and Fatal Prostate Cancer in United States Health Professionals, *Cancer Epidemiology Biomarkers & Prevention,* Vol. 8 (April 1999); 277-282.

31 Enokida, H., et al. "Smoking Influences Aberrant CpG Hypermethylation of Multiple Genes in Human Prostate Carcinoma, *Cancer,* Vol. 106, No. 1 (Dec. 2005); 79-86.

32 Barrett-Connor E., et al. "Cigarette Smoking and Increased Endogenous Estrogen Levels in Men," *American Journal of Epidemiology,* Vol. 126, No. 2 (Aug. 1987); 187-192.

33 Plaskon, L., et al, "Cigarette Smoking and Risk of Prostate Cancer in Middle-Aged Men," *Cancer Epidemiology Biomarkers & Prevention,* Vol. 12 (July 2003); 604-609.

34 Honda, G., et al. "Vasectomy, Cigarette Smoking, and Age at First Sexual Intercourse as Risk Factors for Prostate Cancer in Middle-Aged Men," *British Journal of Cancer,* Vol. 57, No.3 (March 1988); 326-331.

35 McElroy, J., et al. "Cadmium Exposure and Breast Cancer Risk." *Journal of the National Cancer Institute,* Vol. 98, No. 12 (June 2006); 869-873.

36 Elghany, N., et al. "Occupation, Cadmium Exposure, and Prostate Cancer, *Epidemiology,* Vol. 1, No. 2 (March 1990); 107-115.

37 Mills, P.K., et al. "Prostate Cancer Risk in California Farm Workers," *Journal of Occupational and Environmental Medicine,* Vol. 45, No. 3 (March 2003); 249-258.

38 Fleming, L., et al. "Cancer Incidence in a Cohort of Licensed Pesticide Applicators in Florida," *Journal of Occupational and Environmental Medicine,* Vol. 41, No. 4 (April 1999); 279-288.

39 Alavanja, M., et al. "Use of Agricultural Pesticides and Prostate Cancer Risk in the Agricultural Health Study Cohort," *American Journal of Epidemiology,* Vol. 157, No. 9 (May 2003); 800-814.

40 Sharpe, C., et al. "Activities and Exposures During Leisure and Prostate Cancer Risk," *Cancer Epidemiology Biomarkers & Prevention,* Vol. 10, No. 8 (Aug. 2001); 855-860.

41   Giovannucci, E., et al., "A Retrospective Cohort Study of Vasectomy and Prostate Cancer in U.S. Men," *Journal of the American Medical Association,* Vol. 269, No. 7 (Feb. 1993); 878-882.

42   ———. "A Prospective Cohort Study of Vasectomy and Prostate Cancer in U.S. Men," *Journal of the American Medical Association,* Vol. 269, No. 7 (Feb. 1993); 873-877.

43   Honda, G., et al. "Vasectomy, Cigarette Smoking, and Age at First Sexual Intercourse as Risk Factors for Prostate Cancer in Middle-Aged Men," *British Journal of Cancer,* Vol. 57, No.3 (March 1988); 326-331.

44   Stanford, J., et al. "Vasectomy and Risk of Prostate Cancer," *Cancer, Epidemiology Biomarkers & Prevention,* Vol. 8 (Oct. 1999); 881-886.

45   Cox, B., et al. "Vasectomy and Risk of Prostate Cancer," *Journal of the American Medical Association,* Vol. 287 No. 23 (June 2002); 3110-3115.

46   Mo, Z., et al. "Early and Late Long-Term Effects of Vasectomy on Serum Testosterone, Dihydrotestosterone, Luteinizing Hormone and Follicle-Stimulating Hormone Levels," *The Journal of Urology,* Vol. 154, No. 6 (Dec. 1995); 2065-2069.

47   John, E.M., et al, "Vasectomy and Prostate Cancer: Results From a Multiethnic Case-Control Study," *Journal of the National Cancer Institute,* Vol. 87, No. 9 (May 1995); 629-31.

Chapter 5

1   Bonierbale, M.; et al, "The ELIXIR Study: Evaluation of Sexual Dysfunction in 4557 Depressed Patients in France," *Current Medical Research and Opinion,* Vol. 19, No. 2 (March 2003); 114-124.

2   Gregorian, R., et al. "Antidepressant-Induced Sexual Dysfunction," *The Annals of Pharmacotherapy,* Vol. 36, No. 10 (Oct. 2002); 1577-1589.

3   Waldinger, M., et al, "Effect of SSRI Antidepressants on Ejaculation: A Double-Blind, Randomized, Placebo-Controlled Study With Fluoxetine, Fluvoxamine, Paroxetine, and Sertraline," *Journal of Clinical Psychopharmacology,* Vol. 18, No. 4 (Aug. 1998); 274-281.

4   Nurnberg, H., "Managing Treatment-Emergent Sexual Dysfunction Associated with Serotonergic Antidepressants: Before and After Sildenafil, *Journal of Psychiatric Practice,* Vol. 7, No. 2 (March 2001); 92-108.

5   Labbate, L., et al. "Antidepressant-Related Eerectile Dysfunction: Management Via Avoidance, Switching Antidepressants, Antidotes, and Adaptation," *The Journal of Clinical Psychiatry,* Vol. 64, No. 10 (Aug. 2003); 11-9.

6   Kantor, J., et al. "Prevalence of Erectile Dysfunction and Active Depression: An Analytic Cross-Sectional Study of General Medical Patients," *American Journal of Epidemiology,* Vol. 156, No. 11 (Dec. 2002).

7 Bacon, C., et al. "Sexual Function in Men Older Than 50 Years of Age: Results from the Health Professionals Follow-up Study," *Annals of Internal Medicine*, Vol. 139, No. 3 (Aug. 2003); 161-168.

8 Kirby, M., et al. "Is Erectile Dysfunction a Marker for Cardiovascular Disease?" *International Journal of Clinical Practice*, Vol. 55, No.9 (Nov. 2001); 614-618.

9 Billups, K., et al. "Erectile Dysfunction Is a Marker for Cardiovascular Disease: Results of the Minority Health Institute Expert Advisory Panel," *The Journal of Sexual Medicine*, Vol 2, No. 1 (Jan. 2005); 40.

10 Min, J., et al. "Prediction of Coronary Heart Disease by Erectile Dysfunction in Men Referred for Nuclear Stress Testing." *Archives of Internal Medicine*, Vol. 166, No. 2 (Jan. 2006); 201-206.

11 Grover, S., et al. "The Prevalence of Erectile Dysfunction in the Primary Care Setting," *Archives of Internal Medicine*, Vol. 166, No. 2 (Jan. 2006); 213-219.

12 Wei, M., et al, "Total Cholesterol and High Density Lipoprotein Cholesterol as Important Predictors of Erectile Dysfunction," *American Journal of Epidemiology*, Vol. 140, No. 10 (Nov. 1994); 930-937.

13 Saltzman, E., et al. "Improvement in Erectile Function in Men with Organic Erectile Dysfunction by Correction of Elevated Cholesterol Levels: a Clinical Observation," *Journal of Urology*, Vol. 172, No. 1 (July 2004); 255-258.

14 Dhindsa S., et al. "Frequent Occurrence of Hypogonadotropic Hypogonadism in Type 2 Diabetes," *The Journal of Clinical Endocrinology & Metabolism*, Vol. 89, No. 11 (Nov. 2004); 5462-5468.

15 Thompson, I., et al. "Erectile Dysfunction and Subsequent Cardiovascular Disease," *Journal of the American Medical Association*, Vol. 294, No. 23 (Dec. 2005); 2996-3002.

16 Pomeranz, H., et al. "Nonarteritic Ischemic Optic Neuropathy Developing Soon After Use of Sildenafil (Viagra): A Report of Seven New Cases," *Journal of Neuro-Ophthalmology*, Vol. 25, No. 1 (March 2005); 9-13.

17 Fraunfelder, F, et al. "Drug Related Adverse Effects of Clinical Importance to the Opthalmologist," *American Academy of Ophthalmology* (Nov. 2003); 22.

18 Roizenblatt, S., Et al. "A Double-Blind, Placebo-Controlled, Crossover Study of Sildenafil in Obstructive Sleep Apnea," *Archives of Internal Medicine*, Vol. 166, No. 16 (Sept. 2006); 1763-1767.

19 Gilad, R., et al. "Tonic-Clonic Seizures in Patients Taking Sildenafil," *British Medical Journal*, Vol. 325, No. 7 (Oct. 2002); 369:869.

20 Riazi, K., et al. "The Proconvulsant Effect of Sildenafil in Mice: Role of Nitric Oxide-cGMP Pathway," *British Journal of Pharmacology*, Vol. 147, No. 8 (April 2006); 935-943.

21 Striano, P., et al. "Epileptic Seizures Can Follow High Doses of Oral Vardenafil, *British Medical Journal*, Vol. 333, No. 7 (Oct. 2006); 785.

22 Koussa, S., et al. "Epileptic Seizures and Vardenafil," *Revue Neurologique (Paris),* Vol. 162, No. 5 (May 2006); 651-652.

23 Wright, P. J. "Comparison of Phosphodiesterase Type 5 (PDE5) Inhibitors, *International Journal of Clinical Practice,* Vol. 60, No. 8 (Aug. 2006); 967-975.

Chapter 6

1 John, E., et al, "Sun Exposure, Vitamin D Receptor Gene Polymorphisms, and Risk of Advanced Prostate Cancer," *Cancer Research,* Vol. 65, No. 12 (June 2005); 5470-5479.

2 Holick, M.F. "Sunlight and Vitamin D for Bone Health and Prevention of Autoimmune Diseases, Cancers, and Cardiovascular Disease," *American Journal of Clinical Nutrition,* Vol. 80, No. 6 (Dec. 2004); 1678S-1688S.

3 Garland, C., "Sun Avoidance Will Increase Incidence of Cancers Overall," *British Medical Journal,* Vol.327 (Nov. 2003); 1228.

4 Zitterman, A. "Vitamin D in Preventive Medicine: Are We Ignoring the Evidence? *British Journal of Nutrition,* Vol. 89, No. 5 (May 2003); 552-572.

5 Zittermann, A, et al. "Low Vitamin D Status: a Contributing Factor in the Pathogenesis of Congestive Heart Failure?" *Journal of the American College of Cardiology,* Vol. 41, No. 1 (Jan 2003); 105-112.

6 Schwartz, G., et al. "Vitamin D Status and Cancer Incidence and Mortality: Something New Under the Sun," *Journal of the National Cancer Institute,* Vol. 98, No. 7 (April 2006); 428-430.

7 Garland, C., et al. "The Role of Vitamin D in Cancer Prevention," *American Journal of Public Health,* Vol. 96, No. 2 (Feb. 2006); 252-261.

8 Peehl, D., et al. "Pathways Mediating the Growth-Inhibitory Actions of Vitamin D in Prostate Cancer, *Journal of Nutrition,* Vol. 133 (July 2003); 2461S-2469S.

9 Giovannucci, E. et al. "Prospective Study of Predictors of Vitamin D Status and Cancer Incidence and Mortality in Men," *Journal of the National Cancer Institute,* Vol. 98, No. 7 (April 2006); 451-459.

10 Bao, B., et al. "One-Alpha, 25-Dihydroxyvitamin D_3 Inhibits Prostate Cancer Cell Invasion via Modulation of Selective Proteases," *Carcinogenesis,* Vol. 27, No. 1 (Jan. 2006); 32-42.

11 Schleithoff, S., et al. "Vitamin D Supplementation Improves Cytokine Profiles in Patients with Congestive Heart Failure: a Double-Blind, Randomized, Placebo-Controlled Trial," *American Journal of Clinical Nutrition,* Vol. 83, No. 4 April 2006); 754-759.

12 Cigolini, M., et al. "Serum 25-Hydroxyvitamin D3 Concentrations and Prevalence of Cardiovascular Disease Among Type 2 Diabetic Patients," *Diabetes Care,* Vol. 29 (March 2006); 722-724.

13 National Institutes of Health, Dietary Supplement Fact Sheet: Vitamin D, Office of Dietary Supplements, NIH Clinical Center.

14 Rostand, S., et al. "Ultraviolet Light May Contribute to Geographic and Racial Blood Pressure Differences," *Hypertension,* Vol. 30, No. 2 (Aug. 1997); 150-156.

15 Zittermann, A., et al. "Putting Cardiovascular Disease and Vitamin D Insufficiency Into Perspective," *British Journal of Nutrition,* Vol. 94, No. 4 (Oct. 2005); 483-492.

16 Skinner, H., el al. "Vitamin D Intake and the Risk for Pancreatic Cancer in Two Cohort Studies," *Cancer Epidemiology Biomarkers & Prevention,* Vol. 15, (Sept. 2006); 1688-1695.

17 Allain T., et al. "Hypovitaminosis D in Older Adults, *Gerontology,* Vol. 49, No. 5 (Sept.-Oct. 2003); 273-278.

18 Turhimaa, P., et al. "Vitamin D and Prostate Cancer, *The Journal of Steroid Biochemistry and Molecular Biology,* Vol. 76, No. 1-5 (Jan.-Mar. 2001); 125-134.

19 Walker, A., et al. "Cancer Patterns in Three African Populations Compared With the United States Black Population," *The European Journal of Cancer Prevention,* Vol. 2, No. 4 (July 1993); 313-320.

20 Studzinski, G., et al. "Sunlight: Can It Prevent As Well As Cause Cancer? *Cancer Research,* Vol. 55, No. 18 (Sept. 1995); 4014-4022.

21 Morton, R. Jr. "Racial Differences in Adenocarcinoma of the Prostate in North American Men, *Urology,* Vol. 44, No. 5 (Nov. 1994); 637-645.

22 Bodiwala, D., et al. "Susceptibility to Prostate Cancer: Studies on Interactions Between UVR Exposure and Skin Type," *Carcinogenesis,* Vol. 24, No. 4 (April 2003); 711-717.

23 Schwartz, G. "Multiple Sclerosis and Prostate Cancer: What Do Their Similar Geographies Suggest?" *Neuroepidemiology,* Vol. 11, No. 4-6 (1992); 244-254.

24 Hanchette, C., et al. "Geographic Patterns of Prostate Cancer Mortality. Evidence for a Protective Effect of Ultraviolet Radiation," *Cancer,* Vol. 70, No. 12 (Dec. 1992); 2861-2869.

25 Corder, E., et al. "Seasonal Variation in Vitamin D, Vitamin D-Binding Protein, and Dehydroepiandrosterone: Risk of Prostate Cancer in Black and White Men," *Cancer Epidemiology Biomarkers & Prevention,* Vol. 4, No. 6 (Sept. 1995); 655-659.

26 Freedman, D., et al. "Sunlight and Mortality from Breast, Ovarian, Colon, Prostate, and Non-Melanoma Skin Cancer: a Composite Death Certificate Based Case-Control Study," *Occupational & Environmental Medicine,* Vol. 59, No. 4 (April 2002); 257–262.

27 Luscombe, C., et al. "Exposure to Ultraviolet Radiation: Association With Susceptibility and Age at Presentation With Prostate Cancer," *Lancet,* Vol. 358, No. 9282 (Aug. 2001); 641-642.

28 ———. "Outcome in Prostate Cancer Associations With Skin Type and Polymorphism in Pigmentation-Related Genes," *Carcinogenesis,* Vol. 22, No. 9 (Sept. 2001); 1343-1347.

29 Tuohimaa, P., et al. "Both High and Low Levels of Blood Vitamin D are Associated With a Higher Prostate Cancer Risk: a Longitudinal, Nested Case-Control Study in the Nordic Countries," *International Journal of Cancer,* Vol. 108, No. 1 (Jan. 2004); 104-108.

30 Bischoff-Ferrari, H., et al. "Estimation of Optimal Serum Concentrations of 25-Hydroxyvitamin D for Multiple Health Outcomes," *American Journal of Clinical Nutrition,* Vol. 84, No. 1 (July 2006); 18-28.

31 Van den Derghe, G., et al. "Bone Turnover in Prolonged Critical Illness: Effect of Vitamin D," *Journal of Clinical Endocrinology & Metabolism,* Vol. 88, No. 10 (Oct. 2003); 4623-4632.

32 Grau, M.V., et al. "Vitamin D, Calcium Supplementation, and Colorectal Adenomas: Results of a Randomized Trial," *Journal of the National Cancer Institute,* Vol. 95, No. 23 (Dec. 2003); 1765-1771.

33 Rodriguez, C., et al. "Calcium, Dairy Products, and Risk of Prostate Cancer in a Prospective Cohort of United States Men," *Cancer Epidemiology Biomarkers & Prevention,* Vol. 12 (July 2003); 597-603.

34 Konety, B., et al. "Vitamin D in the Prevention and Treatment of Prostate Cancer," *Seminars in Urologic Oncology,* Vol. 17, No. 2 (May 1999); 77-84.

35 Polek, T., et al. "Vitamin D and Prostate Cancer," *Journal of Andrology,* Vol. 23, No. 1 (Jan.-Feb. 2002); 9-17.

36 Blutt, S., et al. "Vitamin D and Prostate Cancer," *Proceedings of the Society for Experimental Biology and Medicine,* Vol. 221, No. 2 (June 1999); 89-98.

37 Peehl, D.M., et al. "The Role of Vitamin D and Retinoids in Controlling Prostate Cancer Progression," *Endocrine-Related Cancer,* Vol. 10, No. 2 (2003); 131-140.

38 Guyton, K., et al. "Vitamin D and Vitamin D Analogs as Cancer Chemopreventive Agents," *Nutrition Reviews,* Vol. 61, No. 7 (July 2003); 227-238.

39 Mercola, J. "Test Values and Treatment for Vitamin D Deficiency," *Mercola Newsletter*, No. 301 (Feb. 2002).

40 Hein, G., Oelzner P. "Vitamin D Metabolites in Rheumatoid Arthritis: Findings-Hypotheses-Consequences," *Z Rheumatology (German),* Vol. 59, No. 1 (2000); 28-32.

41 Timms, P.M., et al. "Circulating MMP9, Vitamin D and Variation in the TIMP-1 Response with VDR Genotype: Mechanisms for Inflammatory Damage in Chronic Disorders," *QJM: An International Journal of Medicine,* Vol. 95, No. 12 (Dec. 2002); 787-796.

42 Houghton, L. A., et al. "The Case Against Ergocalciferol (vitamin D_2) as a Vitamin Supplement," *American Journal of Clinical Nutrition,* Vol. 84, No. 4 (Oct. 2006); 694-697.

43 Welch, H., et al. "Skin Biopsy Rates and Incidence of Melanoma: Population Based Ecological Study," *British Medical Journal*, Vol. 331 (Sept. 2005); 7518.

Chapter 7

1 Fletcher, R. et al. "Vitamins for Chronic Disease Prevention in Adults," *Journal of the American Medical Association*, Vol. 287, No. 23 (June 2002); 3127-3129.

2 Rose, D., et al. "Omega-3 Fatty Acids as Cancer Chemopreventive Agents," *Pharmacology & Therapeutics*, Vol. 83, No. 3 (Sept. 1999); 217-244.

3 Hughes-Fulford, M., et al. "Arachidonic Acid, an Omega-6 Fatty Acid, Induces Cytoplasmic Phospholipase A2 in Prostate Carcinoma Cells," *Carcinogenesis*, Vol. 26, No 9 (May 2005); 1520-1526.

4 ———. "Arachidonic Acid Activates Phosphatidylinositol 3-Kinase Signaling and Induces Gene Expression in Prostate Cancer," *Cancer Research*, Vol. 66 (Feb. 2006); 1427-1433.

5 Brown, M., et al. "Promotion of Prostatic Metastatic Migration Towards Human Bone Marrow Stoma by Omega 6 and its Inhibition by Omega 3 PUFAs," *British Journal of Cancer*, Vol. 94 (March 2006); 842-853.

6 Terry, P., et al. "Fatty Fish Consumption and Risk of Prostate Cancer," *The Lancet*, Vol. 357, No. 9270 (June 2001); 1764-1766.

7 Terry, P., et al. "Intakes of Fish and Marine Fatty Acids and the Risks of Cancers of the Breast and Prostate and of Other Hormone-Related Cancers: a Review of the Epidemiologic Evidence," *American Journal of Clinical Nutrition*, Vol. 77, No. 3 (June 2003); 532-543.

8 Augustsson, K., et al. "A Prospective Study of Intake of Fish and Marine Fatty Acids and Prostate Cancer," *Cancer Epidemiology, Biomarkers & Prevention*, Vol. 12, No. 1 (Jan. 2003); 64-67.

9 Norrish, A., et al. "Prostate Cancer Risk and Consumption of Fish Oils: a Dietary Biomarker-Based Case-Control Study," *British Journal of Cancer*, Vol. 81, No. 7 (Dec. 1999); 1238-1242.

10 Menendez, J., et al, "Effect of Gamma-Linolenic Acid on the Transcriptional Activity of the Her-2/neu (erbB-2) Oncogene," *Journal of the National Cancer Institute*, Vol. 97, No. 21 (Nov. 2005); 1611-1615.

11 Ohno, Y., et al. "Dietary Beta-Carotene and Cancer of the Prostate: a Case-Control Study in Kyoto, Japan," *Cancer Research*, Vol. 48, No. 5 (March 1988); 1331-1336.

12 Mettlin, C., et al. "Beta-Carotene and Animal Fats and Their Relationship to Prostate Cancer Risk, A case-control study," *Cancer*, Vol. 64, No. 3 Aug. 1989); 605-612.

13 James F. Balch, Phyllis Balch, *Prescription for Nutritional Healing*, 3rd ed. (New York: Avery Books, 2000.

[14] Gokce, N, et al. "Long-Term Ascorbic Acid Administration Reverses Endothelial Vasomotor Dysfunction in Patients Wwith Coronary Artery Disease," *Circulation,* Vol. 99, No. 25 (June 1999); 3234-3240.

[15] Duffy, S., et al. "Treatment of Hypertension With Ascorbic Acid," *The Lancet,* Vol. 354, No. 9195 (Dec. 1999); 2048-2049.

[16] ———. "Effect of Ascorbic Acid Treatment on Conduit Vessel Endothelial Dysfunction in Patients with Hypertension," *American Journal of Physiology - Heart and Circulatory Physiology,* Vol. 280, No. 2 (Feb. 2001); H528-534.

[17] Levine, G., et al. "Ascorbic Acid Reverses Endothelial Vasomotor Dysfunction in Patients With Coronary Artery Disease," *Circulation,* Vol. 93, No. 6 (Mar. 1996); 1107-1113.

[18] Huang, H., et al. "Prospective Study of Antioxidant Micronutrients in the Blood and the Risk of Developing Prostate Cancer," *American Journal of Epidemiology,* Vol. 157, No. 4 (Feb. 2003); 335-344.

[19] Venkateswaran, V., et al. "Modulation of Cell Proliferation and Cell Cycle Regulators by Vitamin E in Human Prostate Carcinoma Cell Lines," *Journal of Urology,* Vol. 168, No. 4 (Oct. 2002); 1578-1582.

[20] Heinonen, O., et al. "Prostate Cancer and Supplementation With Alpha-Tocopherol and Beta-Carotene: Incidence and Mortality in a Controlled Trial," *Journal of the National Cancer Institute,* Vol. 90, No. 6 (March 1998); 440-446.

[21] Chan, J., et al. "Supplemental Vitamin E Intake and Prostate Cancer Risk in a Large Cohort of Men in the United States," *Cancer Epidemiology Biomarkers & Prevention,* Vol. 8 (Oct. 1999); 893-899.

[22] Bruno, S., et al. "Faster Plasma Vitamin E Disappearance in Smokers is Normalized by Vitamin C Supplementation," *Free Radical Biology & Medicine,* Vol. 40, No. 4 (Feb. 2006); 689-697.

[23] Zu, K., et al. "Synergy Between Selenium and Vitamin E in Apoptosis Induction is Associated With Activation of Distinctive Initiator Caspases in Human Prostate Cancer Cells," *Cancer Research,* Vol. 63, No. 20 (Oct.2003); 6988-6995.

[24] Ozmen, H., et al. "Comparison of the Concentration of Trace Metals (Ni, Zn, Co, Cu and Se), Fe, Vitamins A, C and E, and Lipid Peroxidation in Patients with Prostate Cancer," *Clinical Chemistry and Laboratory Medicine,* Vol. 44, No. 2 (Feb. 2006); 175-179.

[25] Sigounas, G., et al. "Dl-Alpha-Tocopherol Induces Apoptosis in Erythroleukemia, Prostate, and Breast Cancer Cells," *Nutrition and Cancer,* Vol. 28, No. 1 (May 1997); 30-35.

[26] Gunawardena, K., et al. "Vitamin E and Other Antioxidants Inhibit Human Prostate Cancer Cells Through Apoptosis," *Prostate,* Vol. 44, No. 4 (Sept. 2000); 287-295.

[27] Tomeo, A., et al. "Antioxidant Effects of Tocotrienols in Patients With Hyperlipidemia and Carotid Stenosis," *Lipids,* Vol. 30, No. 12 (Dec. 1995); 1179-83.

[28] Qureshi, A. "Lowering of Serum Cholesterol in Hypercholesterolemic Humans by Tocotrienols," *American Journal of Clinical Nutrition,* Vol. 53 (1991); 1021S-1026S.
[29] Chandan, K. "Tocotrienol: The Natural Vitamin E to Defend the Nervous System, *Annals of the New York Academy of Sciences,* Vol. 1031 (Dec. 2004); 127–142.
[30] Morris, M. et al. "Relation of the Tocopherol Forms to Incident Alzheimer Disease and to Cognitive Change," *American Journal of Clinical Nutrition,* Vol. 81, No. 2) Feb. 2005); 508-514.
[31] Nesaretnam, K., et al. "Effect of Tocotrienols on the Growth of a Human Breast Cancer Cell Line in Culture," *Lipids,* Vol. 30, No. 12 (Dec. 1995); 1139-1143.
[32] Guthrie, N., et al. "Inhibition of Proliferation of Estrogen Receptor-Negative MDA-MB-435 and-Positive MCF-7 Human Breast Cancer Cells by Palm Oil Tocotrienols and Tamoxifen, Alone and in Combination," *Journal of Nutrition,* Vol. 127, No. 3 (March 1997); 544S-548S.
[33] Conte, C., et al. "Gamma-Tocotrienol Metabolism and Antiproliferative Effect in Prostate Cancer Cells," *Annals of the New York Academy of Sciences,* Vol. 1031 (Dec. 2004); 391-394.
[34] Mizushina, Y. et al. "Inhibitory Effect of Tocotrienol on Eukaryotic DNA Polymerase Lambda and Angiogenesis," *Biochemical and Biophysical Research Communications,* Vol. 339, No. 3 (Jan. 2006); 949-955.
[35] Theriault, A., et al. "Tocotrienol: A Review of its Therapeutic Potential," *Clinical Biochemistry,* Vol. 32, No. 5 (July 1999); 309-319.
[36] Moyad, M., et al. "Vitamin E, Alpha- and Gamma-Tocopherol, and Prostate Cancer," *Seminars in Urologic Oncology,* Vol. 17, No. 2 (May 1999); 85-90.
[37] Weinstein, S., et al. "Serum Alpha-Tocopherol and Gamma-Tocopherol in Relation to Prostate Cancer Risk in a Prospective Study," *Journal of the National Cancer Institute,* Vol. 97, No. 5 (March 2005); 396-399.
[38] Moyad, M., "Selenium and Vitamin E Supplements for Prostate Cancer: Evidence or Embellishment," *Urology,* Vol. 59, No. 4 Supplement 1 (April 2002); 9-19.
[39] Prostate Cancer Research Institute. "Basic Facts on Prostate Cancer." *PCRInsights Magazine,* Vol. 4, No. 2 (May 2001).
[40] Das, S., et al. "Cardioprotection With Palm Tocotrienol: Antioxidant Activity of Tocotrienol is Linked With Its Ability to Stabilize Proteasomes," *American Journal of Physiology: Heart and Circulatory Physiology,* Vol. 289, No. 1 (July 2005); H361-H367.
[41] Jiang, C., et al. "Distinct Effects of Methylseleninic Acid Versus Selenite on Apoptosis, Cell Cycle, and Protein Kinase Pathways in DU145 Human Prostate Cancer Cells," *Molecular Cancer Therapeutics,* Vol. 1 (Oct. 2002); 1059-1066.
[42] Dong, Y., et al. "Prostate Specific Antigen Expression Is Down-Regulated by Selenium through Disruption of Androgen Receptor Signaling," *Cancer Research,* Vol. 64 (Jan. 2004); 19-22.

[43] Clark, L., et al. "Decreased Incidence of Prostate Cancer With Selenium Supplementation: Results of a Double-Bblind Cancer Prevention Trial," *British Journal of Urology International,* Vol. 81, No. 5 (May 1998); 730-734.

[44] Duffield-Lillico, A., et al. "Selenium Supplementation, Baseline Plasma Selenium Status and Incidence of Prostate Cancer: an Analysis of the Complete Treatment Period of the Nutritional Prevention of Cancer Trial," *British Journal of Urology International,* Vol. 91, No. 7 (May 2003); 608-612.

[45] Menter, D., et al. "Selenium Effects on Prostate Cell Growth," *Cancer Epidemiology Biomarkers & Prevention,* Vol. 9, No. 11 (Nov. 2000); 1171-1182.

[46] Li, H., et al. "A Prospective Study of Plasma Selenium Levels and Prostate Cancer Risk," *Journal of the National Cancer Institute,* Vol. 96, No. 9 (May 2004); 696-703.

[47] Taylor, P., et al. "Science Peels the Onion of Selenium Effects on Prostate Carcinogenesis," *Journal of the National Cancer Institute,* Vol. 96, No. 9 (May 2004); 645-647.

[48] Gianduzzo, T., et al. "Prostatic and Peripheral Blood Selenium Levels After Oral Supplementation," *Journal of Urology,* Vol. 170, No. 3 (Sept. 2003); 870-873.

[49] Brooks, J., et al. "Plasma Selenium Level Before Diagnosis and the Risk of Prostate Cancer Development," *Journal of Urology,* Vol. 166, No. 6 (Dec. 2001); 2034-2038.

[50] Van den Brandt, P., et al. "Toenail Selenium Levels and the Subsequent Risk of Prostate Cancer," *Cancer Epidemiology Biomarkers & Prevention,* Vol. 12 (Sept. 2003); 866-871.

[51] Yoshizawa, K., et al. "Study of Prediagnostic Selenium Level in Toenails and the Risk of Advanced Prostate Cancer," *Journal of The National Cancer Institute,* Vol. 90, No. 16 (Aug. 1998); 1219-1224.

[52] Helzlsouer, K., et al. "Association Between Alpha-Tocopherol, Gamma-Tocopherol, Selenium, and Subsequent Prostate Cancer," *Journal of the National Cancer Institute,* Vol. 92, No. 24 (Dec. 2000); 2018-2023.

[53] Feng P., et al. "Zinc Induces Mitochondria Apoptogenesis in Prostate Cells," *Molecular Urology,* Vol. 4, No. 1 (Spring 2000); 31-36.

[54] Kristal, A., et al. "Vitamin and Mineral Supplement Use Is Associated with Reduced Risk of Prostate Cancer," *Cancer Epidemiology Biomarkers & Prevention,* Vol. 8 (Oct. 1999); 887-892.

[55] Costello, L., et al. "Novel Role of Zinc in the Regulation of Prostate Citrate Metabolism and Its Implications in Prostate Cancer," *Prostate,* Vol. 35, No. 4 (June 1998); 285-296.

[56] Costello, L., et al. "Testosterone and Prolactin Regulation of Metabolic Genes and Citrate Metabolism of Prostate Epithelial Cells," *Hormone and Metabolic Research,* Vol. 34, No. 8 (Aug. 2002); 417-424.

57 Fortes C., "The Effect of Zinc and Vitamin A Supplementation on Immune Response in an Older Population," *Journal of the American Geriatrics Society,* Vol.46, No. 1 (Jan. 1998); 19-26.

58 Leitzmann, M., et al. "Zinc Supplement Use and Risk of Prostate Cancer," *Journal of the National Cancer Institute,* Vol. 95, No. 13 (July 2003); 1004-1007.

59 Costello L., et al. "Zinc Supplement Use and Risk of Prostate Cancer," *Journal of the National Cancer Institute,* Vol. 96, No. 3 (Feb. 2004); 239-240.

60 Krone, C., et al. "Zinc Supplement Use and Risk of Prostate Cancer," *Journal of the National Cancer Institute,* Vol. 95, No. 20 (Oct. 2003).

61 Krone, C., et al. "Cadmium in Zinc-Containing Mineral Supplements," *International Journal of Food Sciences and Nutrition,* Vol. 52, No. 4 (July 2001); 379-382.

62 Pastori, M, et al. "Lycopene in Association with Alpha-Tocopherol Inhibits at Physiological Concentrations Proliferation of Prostate Carcinoma Cells," *Biochemical and Biophysical Research Communications,* Vol. 250, No. 3 (Sept. 1998); 582-585.

63 Giovannucci, E., et al. "Intake of Carotenoids and Retinol in Relation to Rrisk of Prostate Cancer," *Journal of the National Cancer Institute,* Vol. 87, No. 23 (Dec. 1995); 1767-1776.

64 ———. "A Prospective Study of Tomato Products, Lycopene, and Prostate Cancer Risk," *Journal of the National Cancer Institute,* Vol. 94, No. 5 (March 2002); 391-398.

65 Chen, W., et al. "Oxidative DNA Damage in Prostate Cancer Patients Consuming Tomato Sauce-Based Entrees as a Whole-Food Intervention," *Journal of the National Cancer Institute,* Vol. 93, No. 24 (Dec. 2001); 1872-1879.

66 Canene-Adams, K., et al. "The Tomato As a Functional Food," *Journal of Nutrition,* Vol. 135 (May 2005); 1226-1230.

67 Campbell, J., et al. "Tomato Phytochemicals and Prostate Cancer Risk," *Journal of Nutrition,* Vol. 134 (Dec. 2004); 3486S-3492S.

68 Obermüller-Jevic, U., et al. "Lycopene Inhibits the Growth of Normal Human Prostate Epithelial Cells in Vitro," *Journal of Nutrition,* Vol. 133 (Nov. 2003); 3356-3360.

69 Vogt, T., et al. "Serum Lycopene, Other Serum Carotenoids, and Risk of Prostate Cancer in US Blacks and Whites," *American Journal of Epidemiology,* Vol. 155, No. 11 (June 2002); 1023-1032.

70 Gann, P., et al. "Lower Prostate Cancer Risk in Men with Elevated Plasma Lycopene Levels," *Cancer Research,* Vol. 59 (March 1999); 1225-1230.

71 Kucuk, O., et al. "Phase II Randomized Clinical Trial of Lycopene Supplementation Before Radical Prostatectomy," *Cancer Epidemiology, Biomarkers & Prevention,* Vol. 10 (Aug. 2001); 861-868.

72 Carbin, B., et al. "Treatment of Benign Prostatic Hyperplasia with Phytosterols," *British Journal of Urology,* Vol. 66, No. 6 (Dec. 1990); 639-641.

73 Cortés, B., et al. "Acute Effects of High-Fat Meals Enriched With Walnuts or Olive Oil on Postprandial Endothelial Function," *Journal of the American College of Cardiology,* Vol. 48 (Sept. 2006); 1666-1671.

74 Awab, A.B., et al. "Peanuts as a Source of Beta-Sitosterol, a Sterol with Anticancer Properties," *Nutrition and Cancer,* Vol. 36, No. 2 (2000); 238-241.

75 Alper, C.M., et al. "Peanut Consumption Improves Indices of Cardiovascular Disease Risk in Healthy Adults," *Journal of the American College of Nutrition,* Vol. 22, No. 2 (2003); 133-141.

76 Xiao, D., et al. "Allyl Isothiocyanate, a Constituent of Cruciferous Vegetables, Inhibits Proliferation of Human Prostate Cancer Cells by Causing G2/M Arrest and Inducing Apoptosis," *Carcinogenesis,* Vol. 24, No. 5 (May 2003); 891-897.

77 Singh, A., et al. "Sulforaphane Induces Caspase-Mediated Apoptosis in Cultured PC-3 Human Prostate Cancer Cells and Retards Growth of PC-3 Xenografts in Vivo," *Carcinogenesis,* Vol. 25, No. 1 (Jan. 2004); 83-90.

78 Sarkar, F., et al. "Indole-3-Carbinol and Prostate Cancer," *Journal of Nutrition,* Vol. 134, No. 12 (Dec. 2004); 3493S-3498S.

79 Chiao, J., et al. "Ingestion of an Isothiocyanate Metabolite from Cruciferous Vegetables Inhibits Growth of Human Prostate Cancer Cell Xenografts by Apoptosis and Cell Cycle Arrest," *Carcinogenesis,* Vol. 25, No. 8 (Aug. 2004); 1403-1408.

80 Fan, S., et al. "BRCA1 and BRCA2 as Molecular Targets for Phytochemicals Indole-3-Carbinol and Genistein in Breast and Prostate Cancer Cells," *British Journal of Cancer,* Vol. 94, No. 3 (Feb. 2006); 407-426.

81 Joseph, M., et al. "Cruciferous Vegetables, Genetic Polymorphisms in Glutathione S-Transferases m1 and t1, and Prostate Cancer Risk," *Nutrition and Cancer,* Vol. 50, No. 2 (2004); 206-213.

82 Kolonel, L., et al. "Vegetables, Fruits, Legumes and Prostate Cancer: a Multiethnic Case-Control Study," *Cancer Epidemiology Biomarkers & Prevention,* Vol. 9 (Aug. 2000); 795-804.

83 Jain, M., et al. "Plant Foods, Antioxidants, and Prostate Cancer Risk: Findings From Case-Control Studies in Canada," *Nutrition and Cancer,* Vol. 34, No. 2 (1999); 173-184.

84 Kristal, A., et al. "Brassica Vegetables and Prostate Cancer Risk: a Review of the Epidemiological Evidence," *Nutrition and Cancer,* Vol. 42, No. 1 (2002); 1-9.

85 Cohen, J., et al. "Fruit and Vegetable Intakes and Prostate Cancer Risk, *Journal of the National Cancer Institute,* Vol. 92, No. 1 (Jan. 2000); 61-68.

86 Key, T., et al. "Fruits and Vegetables and Prostate Cancer: No Association Among 1,104 cases in a Prospective Study of 130,544 Men in the European Prospective

Investigation into Cancer and Nutrition (EPIC)," *International Journal of Cancer,* Vol. 109, No. 1 (March 2004); 119-124.

[87] Schuurman, A., et al. "Vegetable and Fruit Consumption and Prostate Cancer Risk: a Cohort Study in The Netherlands," *Cancer Epidemiology Biomarkers and Prevention,* Vol. 7, No. 8 (Aug. 1998); 673-680.

[88] Giovannucci, E., et al. "A Prospective Study of Cruciferous Vegetables and Prostate Cancer," *Cancer Epidemiology Biomarkers & Prevention,* Vol. 12 (Dec. 2003); 1403-1409.

[89] Leung, L., et al. "Theaflavins in Black Tea and Catechins in Green Tea are Equally Effective Antioxidants," *Journal of Nutrition,* Vol. 131 (April 2001); 2248-2251.

[90] Hirata, K., et al. "Black Tea Increases Coronary Flow Velocity Reserve in Healthy Male Subjects," *The American Journal of Cardiology,* Vol. 93, No. 11 (June 2004); 1384-1388.

[91] Duffy, J., et al. "Short- and Long-Term Black Tea Consumption Reverses Endothelial Dysfunction in Patients With Coronary Artery Disease," *Circulation,* Vol. 104, No. 2 (July 2001); 151-156.

[92] Jian, L., et al. "Protective Effect of Green Tea Against Prostate Cancer: a Case-Control Study in Southeast China," *International Journal of Cancer,* Vol. 108, No. 1 (Jan. 2004); 130-135.

[93] Weisburger, J., "Tea and Health: the Underlying Mechanisms," *Proceedings of the Society for Experimental Biology and Medicine,* Vol. 220 (1999); 271-275.

[94] Muktar, H., et al. "Green Tea in Chemoprevention of Cancer," *Toxicological Sciences,* Vol. 52 (Supplement) (Dec. 1999); 111-117.

[95] Fang, M., et al. "Tea Polyphenol (-)-Epigallocatechin-3-Gallate Inhibits DNA Methyltransferase and Reactivates Methylation-Silenced Genes in Cancer Cell Lines," *Cancer Research,* Vol. 63 (Nov. 2003); 7563-7570.

[96] Bettuzzi, S., et al. "Chemoprevention of Human Prostate Cancer by Oral Administration of Green Tea Catechins in Volunteers with High-Grade Prostate Intraepithelial Neoplasia: A Preliminary Report from a One-Year Proof-of-Principle Study, *Cancer Research,* Vol. 66, No. 2 (Jan. 2006); 1234-1240.

[97] Sacks, F., et al. "Soy Protein, Isoflavones, and Cardiovascular Health. *Circulation,* Advisory for Professionals From the Nutrition Committee, Published online Jan. 17, 2006.

[98] Xiang, H., et al. "A Comparative Study of Growth-Inhibitory Effects of Isoflavones and Their Metabolites on Human Breast and Prostate Cancer Cell Lines," *Nutrition and Cancer,* Vol. 42, No. 2 (2002); 224-32.

[99] Brooks, J., et al. "Supplementation With Flaxseed Alters Estrogen Metabolism in Postmenopausal Women to a Greater Extent Than Does Supplementation with an Equal Amount of Soy," *American Journal of Clinical Nutrition,* Vol. 79, No. 2 (Feb. 2004); 318-325.

[100] Demark-Wahnefried W., et al. "Pilot Study of Dietary Fat Restriction and Flaxseed Supplementation in Men with Prostate Cancer Before Surgery: Exploring the Effects on Hormonal Levels, Prostate-Specific Antigen, and Histopathologic Features," *Urology,* Vol. 58, No. 1 (July 2001); 47-52.

[101] Leitzmann, M., et al. "Dietary Intake of Omega–3 and Omega–6 Fatty Acids and the Risk of Prostate Cancer," *American Journal of Clinical Nutrition,* Vol. 80, No. 1 (July 2004); 204-216.

Chapter 8

[1] Hedelin, M., et al. "Dietary Phytoestrogen, Serum Enterolactone and Risk of Prostate Cancer: The Cancer Prostate Sweden Study (Sweden)," *Cancer Causes and Control,* Vol. 17, No. 2 (March 2006); 169-180.

[2] Adlercreutz, H., et al. "Phytoestrogens and Prostate Disease," *Journal of Nutrition,* Vol. 130, No. 5 (July 2000); 658S-659S.

[3] *Alternative Medicine Review,* "Plant Sterols and Sterolins," Vol. 6, No. 2 (April 2001); 203-206.

[4] Thompson, G. R., et al. "History and Development of Plant Sterol and Stanol Esters for Cholesterol-Lowering Purposes," *The American Journal of Cardiology,* Vol. 96 No. 1A (July 2005); 3D-9D.

[5] Katan, M.B., et al. "Efficacy and Safety of Plant Stanols and Sterols in the Management of Blood Cholesterol Levels," *Mayo Clinic Proceedings,* Vol. 78 No. 8 (Aug. 2003); 965-978.

[6] Nguyen, T. "The Cholesterol-Lowering Action of Plant Stanol Esters," *Journal of Nutrition,* Vol. 129 (Dec. 1999); 2109-2112.

[7] Gilliver, S.C., et al. "Androgens Modulate the Inflammatory Response During Acute Wound Healing," *Journal of Cell Science,* Vol. 119 (Jan. 2006); 722-732.

[8] Gerber, G. S., et al. "Randomized, Double-Blind, Placebo-Controlled Trial of Saw Palmetto in Men with Lower Urinary Tract Symptoms," *Urology,* Vol. 58, No. 6 (Dec. 2001); 960-964.

[9] Plosker, G. L., et al. "Serenoa Repens (Permixon). A Review of Its Pharmacology and Therapeutic Efficacy in Benign Prostatic Hyperplasia," *Drugs & Aging,* Vol. 9, No. 5 (Nov. 1996); 379-395.

[10] Pytel, Y.A., et al. "Long-Term Clinical and Biologic Effects of the Lipidosterolic Extract of Serenoa Repens in Patients with Symptomatic Benign Prostatic Hyperplasia," *Advances in Therapy,* Vol. 19, No. 6 (Nov.-Dec. 2002); 297-306.

[11] Marks, L., et al. "Effects of a Saw Palmetto Herbal Blend in Men With Symptomatic Benign Prostatic Hyperplasia," *The Journal of Urology,* Vol. 163, No. 5 (May 2000); 1451-1456.

12 Wilt, T. J., et al. "Saw Palmetto Extracts for Treatment of Benign Prostatic Hyperplasia," *Journal of the American Medical Association,* Vol. 280 No. 18 (Nov. 1998); 1604-1609.

13 Boyle, P., et al. "Updated Meta-Analysis of Clinical Trials of Serenoa Repens Extract in the Treatment of Symptomatic Benign Prostatic Hyperplasia," *British Journal of Urology International,* Vol. 93 No. 6 (April 2004); 751.

14 Ishani, A., et al. "Pygeum Africanum for the Treatment of Patients With Benign Prostatic Hyperplasia: a Systematic Review and Quantitative Meta-analysis," *The American Journal of Medicine,* Vol. 109, No. 8 (Dec. 2000); 654-664.

15 Breza, J., et al. "Efficacy and Acceptability of Tadenan (Pygeum Africanum Extract) in the Treatment of Benign Prostatic Hyperplasia (BPH): a Multicentre Trial in Central Europe," *Current Medical Research and Opinion,* Vol. 14, No. 3 (1998); 127-139.

16 Bartlet, A., et al. "Efficacy of Pygeum Africanum Extract in the Medical Therapy of Urination Disorders Due to Benign Prostatic Hyperplasia: Evaluation of Objective and Subjective Parameters. A Placebo-Controlled Double-Blind Multicenter Study," *Wiener klinische Wochenschrift,* Vol. 102, No. 22 (Nov. 1990); 667-673.

17 Schleich, S., et al. "Activity-Guided Isolation of an Antiandrogenic Compound of Pygeum Africanum," *Planta Medica,* Vol. 72 (April 2006); 547-551.

18 Wilt, T. "Pygeum Africanum for Benign Prostatic Hyperplasia," *Cochrane Review* (July 2006).

19 Yablonsky, F., et al. "Antiproliferative Effect of Pygeum Africanum Extract on Rat Prostatic Fibroblasts," *The Journal of Urology,* Vol. 157, No. 6 (June 1997); 2381-2387.

20 Hryb, D. J., et al. "The Effect of Extracts of the Roots of the Stinging Nettle (Urtica Dioica) on the Interaction of SHBG With Its Receptor on Human Prostatic Membranes," *Planta Medica,* Vol. 61, No. 1 (Feb. 1995); 31-32.

21 Schottner, M., et al. "Lignans From the Roots of Urtica Dioica and Their Metabolites Bind to Human Sex Hormone Binding Globulin (SHBG)," *Planta Medica,* Vol. 63 No. 6 (Dec. 1997); 529–532.

22 Hirano, T., et al. "Effects of Stinging Nettle Root Extracts and Their Steroidal Components on the Na+,K(+)-ATPase of the Benign Prostatic Hyperplasia," *Planta Medica,* Vol 60 No. 1 (Feb. 1994); 30-33.

23 Schneider, T., et al. "Stinging Nettle Root Extract (Bazoton-Uno) in Long Term Treatment of Benign Prostatic Syndrome (BPS). Results of a Randomized, Double-Blind, Placebo Controlled Multicenter Study After 12 Months," *Der Urologe.* (German Urology), Vol. 43, No. 3 March 2004); 302-306.

24 Konrad, L., et al. "Antiproliferative Effect on Human Prostate Cancer Cells by a Stinging Nettle Root (Urtica Dioica) Extract," *Planta Medica,* Vol. 66, No. 1 (Feb. 2000); 44-447.

25 Lichius, J. J., et al. "The Inhibiting Effects of Components of Stinging Nettle Roots on Experimentally Induced Prostatic Hyperplasia in Mice," *Planta Medica*, Vol. 5, No. 7 (Oct. 1999); 666-668.

26 Dutkiewicz, S. "Usefulness of Cernilton in the Treatment of Benign Prostatic Hyperplasia," *International Urology and Nephrology*, Vol. 28, No.1 (1996); 49-53.

27 MacDonald, R., et al. "A Systematic Review of Cernilton for the Treatment of Benign Prostatic Hyperplasia," *British Journal of Urology International*, Vol. 85, No. 7 (May 2000); 836-841.

28 Wilt, T., et al. "Cernilton for Benign Prostatic Hyperplasia," *Cochrane Database of Systematic Review* (2000).

29 Buck, A.C., et al. "Treatment of Outflow Tract Obstruction Due to Benign Prostatic Hyperplasia with the Pollen Extract, Cernilton. A Double-Blind, Placebo-Controlled Study," *British Journal of Urology*, Vol. 66 (1990); 398-404.

30 Yasumoto, R., et al. "Clinical Evaluation of Long-Term Treatment Using Cernitin Pollen Extract in Patients with Benign Prostatic Hyperplasia," *Clinical Therapeutics*, Vol. 17, No. 1 (Jan.-Feb. 1995); 82-87.

31 Rugendorff, E.W., et al. "Results of Treatment With Pollen Extract (Cernilton N) in Chronic Prostatitis and Prostatodynia," *British Journal of Urology*, Vol 71, No. 4 (April 1993); 433-438.

32 Habib, F.K., et al. "Identification of a Prostate Inhibitory Substance in a Pollen Extract," *The Prostate*, Vol. 26, No. 3 (March 1995); 133-139.

33 Habib, F.K., et al. "In Vitro Evaluation of the Pollen Extract, Cernitin T-60, in the Regulation of Prostate Cell Growth," *British Journal of Urology*, Vol. 66, No. 4 (Oct. 1990), 398-397.

34 Zhang, X., et al. "Isolation and Characterization of a Cyclic Hydroxamic Acid From a Pollen Extract, Which Inhibits Cancerous Cell Growth in Vitro," *Journal of Medical Chemistry*, Vol. 38, No. 4 (Feb. 1995); 735-738.

35 Li, M., et al. "Antitumor Activity of Z-Ajoene, a Natural Compound Purified from Garlic: Antimitotic and Microtubule-Interaction Properties," *Carcinogenesis*, Vol. 23, No. 4 (April 2002); 573-579.

36 Pinto, J., et al. "Antiproliferative Effects of Allium Derivatives from Garlic," *Journal of Nutrition*, Vol. 131 (2001); 1058S-1060S.

37 Xiao, D., et al. "Diallyl Trisulfide, a Constituent of Processed Garlic, Inactivates Akt to Trigger Mitochondrial Translocation of BAD and Caspase-Mediated Aapoptosis in Human Prostate Cancer Cells," *Carcinogenesis*, Vol. 27, No. 3 (March 2006); 533-540.

38 Pinto, J., et al. "Alterations of Prostate Biomarker Expression and Testosterone Utilization in Human LNCaP Prostatic Carcinoma Cells by Garlic-Derived S-Allylmercaptocysteine," *The Prostate*, Vol. 45, No. 4 (Dec. 2000); 304-314.

[39] Hsing, A., et al. "Allium Vegetables and Risk of Prostate Cancer: A Population-Based Study," *Journal of the National Cancer Institute,* Vol. 94, No. 21 (Nov. 2002); 1648-1651.

[40] Pedraza-Chaverrí, J., et al. "Garlic Prevents Hypertension Induced by Chronic Inhibition of Nitric Oxide Synthesis," *Life Sciences,* Vol. 62, No. 6 (Jan. 1998); 71-77.

[41] Borek, C. "Garlic Reduces Dementia and Heart-Disease Risk," *The Journal of Nutrition,* Vol. 136 (March 2006); 810S-812S.

[42] Ashton, A.K., et al. "Antidepressant-Induced Sexual Dysfunction and Ginkgo Biloba," *American Journal of Psychiatry,* Vol. 157 (May 2000); 836-837.

[43] Cohen, A.J., et al. "Ginkgo Biloba for Antidepressant-Induced Sexual Dysfunction," *Journal of Sex & Marital Therapy,* Vol. 24, No. 2 (April-June 1998); 139-143.

[44] Pretner, E., et al. "Cancer-Related Overexpression of the Peripheral-typeBenzodiazepine Receptor and Cytostatic Anticancer Effects of Ginkgo Biloba Extract," *Anticancer Research,* Vol. 26, No. 1A (Jan.-Feb. 2006).

[45] Yoshikawa, T., et al. "Ginkgo Biloba Leaf Extract: Review of Biological Actions and Clinical Applications," *Antioxidants and Redox Signaling,* Vol. 1, No. 4 (Winter 1999); 469-480.

[46] Le Bars, P.L., et al. "Efficacy and Safety of a Ginkgo Biloba Extract," *Public Health and Nutrition.* Vol. 3 No. 4A (Dec. 2000); 495-499.

[47] Berges R. R., et al. "Randomized, Placebo-Controlled Double Blind Clinical Trial of B-Sitosterol in Patients with Benign Prostatic Hyperplasia," *The Lancet,* Vol. 345, No. 8964 (June 1995); 1529-1532.

[48] Berges, R. R., et al. "Treatment of Symptomatic Benign Prostatic Hyperplasia with B-Sitosterol: an 18-Month Follow-Up," *British Journal of Urology International,* Vol. 85, No. 7 (May 2000); 842-846.

[49] Wilt, T. J., et al. "Beta-Sitosterols for Benign Prostatic Hyperplasia," *Cochrane Database of Systematic Reviews* (online), No. 2 (2000).

[50] Klippel, K. F., et al. "A Multicentric, Placebo-Controlled, Double-Blind Clinical Trial of Beta-Sitosterol (Phytosterol) for the Treatment of Benign Prostatic Hypertrophy," (German BPH-Phyto Study Group) *British Journal of Urology,* Vol. 80, No. 3 (Sept. 1997); 427-432.

[51] Pienta, K. J., et al. "Inhibition of Spontaneous Metastasis in a Rat Prostate Cancer Model by Oral Administration of Modified Citrus Pectin," *Journal of the National Cancer Institute,* Vol. 87, No. 5 (March 1995); 348-353.

[52] Nangia-Makker, P., et al. "Inhibition of Human Cancer Cell Growth and Metastasis in Nude Mice by Oral Intake of Modified Citrus Pectin," *Journal of the National Cancer Institute,* Vol. 94, No. 24 (Dec. 2002); 1854-1862.

[53] Strum, S. B., et al. "Modified Citrus Pectin Slows PSA Doubling Time: a Pilot Clinical Trial. Presented at the International Conference on Diet and Prevention of Cancer. Tampere, Finland (May 28-June 2, 1999).

[54] Guess, B. W., et al. "Modified Citrus Pectin (MCP) Increases the Prostate-Specific Antigen Doubling Time in Men with Prostate Cancer: a Phase II Pilot Study," *Prostate Cancer and Prostatic Diseases,* Vol. 6, No. 4 (Dec. 2003); 301-304.

[55] Wilt, T. J., et al. "Phytotherapy for Benign Prostatic Hyperplasia," *Public Health Nutrition,* Vol. 3, No 4A (Dec. 2000); 459-472.

[56] Krzeski, T., et al. "Combined Extracts of Urtica Dioica and Pygeum Africanum in the Treatment of Benign Prostatic Hyperplasia: Double-Blind Comparison of Two Doses," *Clinical Therapeutics,* Vol. 15, No. 6 (Nov.-Dec. 1993); 1011-1020.

[57] Hartmann, R.W., et al. "Inhibition of 5 Alpha-Reductase and Aromatase by PHL-00801 (Prostatonin®), a Combination of PY 102 (Pygeum Africanum) and UR 102 (Urtica Dioica) Extracts," *Phytomedicine,* Vol. 3, No. 2 (March 1996); 121-128.

[58] Preuss, H.G., et al. "Randomized Trial of a Combination of Natural Products (Cernitin, Saw Palmetto, B-Sitosterol, Vitamin E) on Symptoms of Benign Prostatic Hyperplasia (BPH)," *International Urology and Nephrology,* Vol. 33, No. 2 (June 2001); 217-225.

[59] Koch, E. "Extracts From Fruits of Saw Palmetto (Sabal Serrulata) and Roots of Stinging Nettle (Urtica Dioica): Viable Alternatives in the Medical Treatment of Benign Prostatic Hyperplasia and Associated Lower Urinary Tracts Symptoms," *Planta Medica,* Vol. 67, No. 6 (Aug. 2001); 489-500.

[60] Lopatkin, N., et al. "Long-Term Efficacy and Safety of a Combination of Sabal and Urtica Extract for Lower Urinary Tract Symptoms: a Placebo-Controlled, Double-Blind, Multicenter Trial," *World Journal of Urology* (June 2005).

[61] Preuss, H. G., et al. "Randomized Trial of a Combination of Natural Products (Cernitin, Saw Palmetto, B-Sitosterol, Vitamin E) on Symptoms of Benign Prostatic Hyperplasia (BPH)," *International Urology and Nephrology,* Vol. 33, No. 2 (June 2001); 217-225.

[62] Wilt, T., et al. "Serenoa Repens for Benign Prostatic Hyperplasia," *Cochrane Database of Systematic Reviews,* Vol. 3 (2002); CD001423.

[63] Goetzl, M., et al. "Finasteride as a Chemopreventive Agent in Prostate Cancer: Impact of the Prostate Cancer Prevention Trial on Urologic Practice," *Nature Clinical Practice Urology,* Vol. 3, No. 8 (Sept. 2006).

Chapter 9

[1] Kirby, M., et al. "Endothelial Dysfunction Links Erectile Dysfunction to Heart Disease," *International Journal of Clinical Practice*, Vol. 59, No. 2 (Feb. 2005); 225-229.

[2] Hallemeesch, M., et al. "Reduced Arginine Availability and Nitric Oxide Production," Clinical Nutrition, Vol. 21, No. 4 (Aug. 2002); 273-279.

[3] Burnett, A. L. "Role of Nitric Oxide in the Physiology of Erection," *Biology of Reproduction,* Vol. 52, No. 3 (March 1995); 485-489.

[4] Choi, Y.D., et al. "The Distribution of Nitric Oxide Synthase in Human Corpus Cavernosum on Various Impotent Patients," *Yonsei Medical Journal,* Vol. 38, No. 3 (June 1997); 125-132.

[5] Huynh, N., et al. "Amino Acids, Arginase and Nitric Oxide in Vascular Health," *Clinical and Experimental Pharmacology and Physiology,* Vol. 33, No. 1-2 (Jan. 2006); 1.

[6] Stuehr, D. "Enzymes of the L-Arginine to Nitric Oxide Pathway," *The Journal of Nutrition,* Vol. 134 (Oct. 2004); 2748S-2751S.

[7] Morris, S. "Enzymes of Arginine Metabolism," *The Journal of Nutrition,* Vol. 134 (Oct. 2004); 2743S-2747S.

[8] Zorgniotti, A.W., et al. "Effect of Large Doses of the Nitric Oxide Precursor, L-Arginine, on Erectile Dysfunction," *International Journal of Impotence Research,* Vol. 6, No.1 (March 1994); 33-35.

[9] Chen, J., et al. "Effect of Oral Administration of High-Dose Nitric Oxide Donor L-Arginine in Men with Organic Erectile Dysfunction: Results of a Double-Blind, Randomized, Placebo-Controlled Study," *British Journal of Urology International,* Vol. 83 (Feb. 1999); 269.

[10] Ito, T., et al. "The Effects of ArginMax, a Natural Dietary Supplement for Enhancement of Male Sexual Function," *Hawaii Medical Journal,* Vol. 57, No. 12 (Dec. 1998); 741-744.

[11] Clarkson, P., et al. "Oral L-Arginine Improves Endothelium-Dependent Dilation in Hypercholesterolemic Young Adults," *The Journal of Clinical Investigation,* Vol. 97, No. 8 (April 1996); 1989-1994.

[12] Doutreleau, S., et al. "Chronic L-Arginine Supplementation Enhances Endurance Exercise Tolerance in Heart Failure Patients," *International Journal of Sports Medicine,* Vol. 27, No. 7 (July 2006); 567-572.

[13] Broeders, A.W., et al. "Hypercholesterolemia Enhances Thromboembolism in Arterioles but Not Venules: Complete Reversal by L-Arginine," *Arteriosclerosis, Thrombosis, and Vascular Biology,* Vol. 22, No. 4 (April 2002); 680-685.

[14] Broeders, A.W., et al. "Endogenous Nitric Oxide Protects Against Thromboembolism in Venules But Not in Arterioles," *Arteriosclerosis, Thrombosis, and Vascular Biology,* Vol. 18 (1998); 139-145.

[15] Stokes, G. S., et al. "Interactions of L-Arginine, Isosorbide Mononitrate, and Angiotensin II Inhibitors on Arterial Pulse Wave," *American Journal of Hypertension,* Vol. 16, No. 9 Pt 1 (Sept. 2003); 719-724.

[16] Fenning, A., et al. "L-Arginine Attenuates Cardiovascular Impairment in DOCA-Salt Hypertensive Rats," *American Journal of Physiology:Heart and Circulatory Physiology,* Vol 289 (May 2005); H1408-H1416.

[17] Susic, D., et al. "Prolonged L-Arginine on Cardiovascular Mass and Myocardial Hemodynamics and Collagen in Aged Spontaneously Hypertensive Rats and Normal Rats," *Hypertension,* Vol. 33, No. 1 (Jan. 1999); 451-455.

[18] ———. "Isolated Systolic Hypertension in Elderly WKY Is Reversed With L-Arginine and ACE Inhibition," *Hypertension*, Vol. 38, No. 6 (Dec. 2001); 1422.

[19] Hayashi, T., et al. "L-Citrulline and L-Arginine Supplementation Retards the Progression of High-Cholesterol-Diet-Induced Atherosclerosis in Rabbits," *Proceedings of the National Academy of Sciences of the United States of America*, Vol. 102, No. 38 (Sept. 2005); 13681-13686.

[20] Bivalacqua, T., et al. "Endothelial Dysfunction in Erectile Dysfunction: Role of the Endothelium in Erectile Physiology and Disease," *Journal of Andrology*, Vol. 24, No. 6 Supplement (Nov.-Dec. 2003).

[21] Hecker, M., et al. "The Metabolism of L-Arginine and Its Significance for the Biosynthesis of Endothelium-Derived Relaxing Factor: Cultured Endothelial Cells Recycle L- Citrulline to L-Arginine," *Proceedings of the National Academy of Sciences of the United States of America*, Vol. 87 (1990); 8612-8616.

[22] Brosnan, M., et al. "Renal Arginine Metabolism," *The Journal of Nutrition*, Vol. 134 (Oct. 2004); 2791S-2795S.

[23] Waugh, W., et al. "Oral Citrulline as Arginine Precursor May Be Beneficial in Sickle Cell Disease: Early Phase Two Results," *Journal of the National Medical Association*, Vol. 93, No. 10 (Oct. 2001); 363-371.

[24] Riazi, K., et al. "The Proconvulsant Effect of Sildenafil in Mice: Role of Nitric Oxide-cGMP Pathway," *British Journal of Pharmacology*, Vol. 147, No. 8 (April 2006); 935-943.

[25] Stanislavov, R., et al. "Treatment of Erectile Dysfunction with Pycnogenol and L-arginine," *Journal of Sex & Marital Therapy*, Vol. 29, No. 3 (May-June 2003); 207-213.

[26] Susset, J. G., et al. "Effect of Yohimbine Hydrochloride on Erectile Impotence: a Double-Blind Study," *Journal of Urology*, Vol. 141, No. 6 (June 1989); 1360-1363.

[27] Morales, A., et al. "Is Yohimbine Effective in the Treatment of Organic Impotence? Results of a Controlled Trial," *Journal of Urology*, Vol. 137, No. 6 (June 1987); 1168-1172.

[28] Guay, A., et al. "Yohimbine Treatment of Organic Erectile Dysfunction in a Dose-Escalation Trial," *International Journal of Impotence Research*, Vol. 14, No. 1 (Feb. 2002); 25-31.

[29] Pittler, M. H., "Yohimbine in Therapy of Erectile Dysfunction," *Fortschritte der Medizin*, Vol. 116, No.1 (Jan. 1998); 32-33.

[30] James F. Balch, Phyllis Balch, *"Prescription for Nutritional Healing*, 3rd ed., (New York: Avery Books, 2000).

[31] Duke, J. *The Green Pharmacy* (New York: St. Martins Press, 2001).

[32] Murray, M. and Pizzorno, J. *Encylopedia of Natural Medicine*, 2nd Ed, (Rocklin, CA: Prima Publishing, 1998.)

[33] Betz, J. M., et al. "Gas Chromatographic Determination of Yohimbine in Commercial Yohimbe Products," *Journal of the Association of Official Analytical Chemistry International*, Vol. 78, No. 5 (Aug. 1996); 1189-1194.

[34] Waynberg, J., "Aphrodisiacs: Contributions to the Clinical Validation of the Traditional Use of Ptychopetalum Guyanna. Presented at The First International Congress on Ethnopharmacology, Strasbourg, France (June 5-9 1990).

[35] Waynberg, J., "Male Sexual Asthenia - Interest in a Traditional Plant-Derived Medication," *Journal of Ethnopharmacology*, Vol. 45, No. 3 (March 1995).

[36] Salvati, G., et al. "Effects of Panax Ginseng Saponins on Male Fertility," *Panminerva Medica*, Vol 38, No. 4 (Dec. 1996); 249-254.

[37] Choi, Y.D., et al. "In Vitro and in Vivo Experimental Effect of Korean Red Ginseng on Erection," *Journal of Urology*, Vol. 162, No. 4 (Oct. 1999); 1508-1511.

[38] Fahim, M.S., et al. "Effect of Panax Ginseng on Testosterone Level and Prostate in Male Rats," *Archives of Andrology*, Vol. 8, No. 4 (June 1982); 261-263.

[39] Aphale, A., et al. "Subacute Toxicity Study of the Combination of Ginseng (Panax Ginseng) and Ashwagandha (Withania Somnifera) in Rats: a Safety Assessment," *Indian Journal of Physiology and Pharmacology*, Vol. 42, No. 2 (April 1998); 299-302.

[40] Castleman, M. *The New Healing Herbs* (New York: Bantam Books, 2002).

[41] Kim, S., et al. "Ginsenoside-Rs4, a New Type of Ginseng Saponin Concurrently Induces Apoptosis and Selectively Elevates Protein Levels of p53 and p21WAF1 in Human Hepatoma SK-HEP-1 Cells," *European Journal of Cancer*, Vol. 35, No. 3 (March 1999); 507-511.

[42] ―――. "Ginsenoside-Rs3, a New Diol-Type Ginseng Saponin, Selectively Elevates Protein Levels of p53 and p21WAF1 Leading to Induction of Apoptosis in SK-HEP-1 Cells," *Anticancer Research*, Vol. 19, No. 1A (Jan.-Feb. 1999); 487-491.

[43] Oh, M., et al. "Anti-Proliferating Effects of Ginsenoside Rh2 on MCF-7 Human Breast Cancer Cells," *International Journal of Oncology*, Vol. 14, No. 5 (May 1999); 869-875.

[44] Xiaoguang, C., et al. "Cancer Chemopreventive and Therapeutic Activities of Red Ginseng," *Journal of Ethnopharmacology*, Vol. 60, No. 1 (Feb. 1998); 71-78.

[45] Yun T.K., et al. "Non-Organ Specific Cancer Prevention of Ginseng: a Prospective Study in Korea," *International Journal of Epidemiology*, Vol. 27, No. 3 (June 1998); 359-364.

[46] Yun, T.K. "Experimental and Epidemiological Evidence on Non-Organ Specific Cancer Preventive Effect of Korean Ginseng and Identification of Active Compounds," *Mutatation Research*, Vol. 523-524 (Feb.-Mar. 2003); 63-74.

[47] Yuan, C. S., et al. "Brief Communication: American Ginseng Reduces Warfarin's Effect in Healthy Patients," *Annals of Internal Medicine*, Vol. 141, No. 1 (July 2004); 23-27.

48 Gonzales, G. F., et al. "Effect of Lepidium Meyenii (Maca), a Root With Aphrodisiac and Fertility-Enhancing Properties, on Serum Reproductive Hormone Levels in Adult Healthy Men," *The Journal of Endocrinology*, Vol.176, No. 1 (Jan. 2003); 163-168.

49 Zheng, B. L., et al. "Effect of a Lipidic Extract from Lepidium Meyenii on Sexual Behavior in Mice and Rats," *Urology*, Vol. 55, No. 4 (April 2000); 598-602.

50 Cicero, A. F., et al. "Lepidium Meyenii Walp. Improves Sexual Behaviour in Male Rats Independently From Its Action on Spontaneous Locomotor Activity," *Journal of Ethnopharmacology*, Vol. 75, No. 2-3 (May 2001); 225-229.

51 Gonzales, G. F., et al. "Effect of Lepidium Meyenii (Maca) Roots on Spermatogenesis of Male Rats," *Asian Journal of Andrology*, Vol 3, No. 3 (Sept. 2001); 231-233.

52 ———. "Effect of Lepidium Meyenii (MACA) on Sexual Desire and Its Absent Relationship With Serum Testosterone Levels in Adult Healthy Men," *Andrologia*, Vol. 34, No. 6 (Dec. 2002); 367-372.

53 ———. "Lepidium Meyenii (Maca) Improved Semen Parameters in Adult Men," *Asian Journal of Andrology*, Vol. 3, No. 4 (Dec. 2001); 301-303.

54 ———. "Effect of Lepidium Meyenii (Maca) on Spermatogenesis in Male Rats Acutely Exposed to High Altitude (4340 m)," *The Journal of Endocrinology*, Vol. 180, No. 1 (Jan 2004); 87-95.

55 Cui, B., et al. "Imidazole Alkaloids from Lepidium Meyenii," *Journal of Natural Products*, Vol. 66, No. 8 (Aug. 2003); 1101-1103.

56 Kuang, A. K., et al. "Effects of Yang-Restoring Herb Medicines on the Levels of Plasma Corticosterone, Testosterone and Triiodothyronine," *Zhong Xi Yi Jie He Za Zhi (Chinese Journal of Modern Developments in Traditional Medicine)*, Vol. 9, No. 12 (Dec. 1989); 737-738, 710.

57 Tian, L., et al. "Effects of Icariin on the Erectile Function and Expression of Nitrogen Oxide Synthase Isoforms in Corpus Cavernosum of Arterigenic Erectile Dysfunction Rat Model," *Zhonghua yi xue za zhi (Chinese Medical Journal; Free China ed.)*, Vol. 84, No. 11 (June 2004); 954-957.

58 Liao, H. J., et al. "Effect of Epimedium Sagittatum on Quality of Life and Cellular Immunity in Patients of Hemodialysis Maintenance," *Zhongguo Zhong Xi Yi Jie He Za Zhi (Chinese Journal of Integrated Traditional and Western Medicine)*, Vol. 15, No. 4 (April 1995); 202-204.

59 Cai, D., et al. "Clinical and Experimental Research of Epimedium Brevicornum in Relieving Neuroendocrino-Immunological Effect Inhibited By Exogenous Glucocorticoid," *Zhongguo Zhong Xi Yi Jie He Za Zhi (Chinese Journal of Integrated Traditional and Western Medicine)*, Vol. 18, No. 1 (Jan. 1998); 4-7.

60 Chen, X., et. al. "Effects of Epimedium Sagittatum on Soluble IL-2 Receptor and IL-6 Levels in Patients Undergoing Hemodialysis," *Chung HuaNei Ko Tsa Chin (Chinese Journal of Internal Medicine)*, Vol. 34, No. 2 Feb. 1995); 102-104.

[61] Antonio, J., et al. "The Effects of Tribulus Terrestris on Body Composition and Exercise Performance in Resistance-Trained Males," *International Journal of Sport Nutrition and Exercise Metabolism,* Vol. 10, No. 2 (June 2000); 208-215.

[62] Kumanov, F., et al. "Clinical Trial of the Drug "Tribestan," *Savr Med.,* Vol. 4 (1982); 211-215.

[63] Gauthaman, K., "Aphrodisiac Properties of Tribulus Terrestris Extract (Protodioscin) in Normal and Castrated Rats," *Life Sciences,* Vol. 71, No. 12 (Aug. 2002); 1385-1396.

[64] Sharifi , A. M, et al. "Study of Antihypertensive Mechanism of Tribulus Terrestris in 2K1C Hypertensive Rats: Role of Tissue ACE Activity," *Life Sciences,* Vol. 73, No. 23 (Oct. 2003); 2963-2971.

[65] Adimoelja, A., "Phytochemicals and the Breakthrough of Traditional Herbs in the Management of Sexual Dysfunctions," *International Journal of Andrology,* Vol. 23, Supp. 2 (2000); 82-84.

[66] Adaikan, P.G., et al. "Proerectile Pharmacological Effects of Tribulus Terrestris Extract on the Rabbit Corpus Cavernosum," *Annals of the Academy of Medicine, Singapore*; 29(1) (Jan. 2000); 22–26.

[67] Xu, Y.X., et al. "Three New Saponins From Tribulus Terrestris," *Planta Medica,* Vol. 66, No. 6 (Aug. 2000); 545-550.

[68] Kostove, I., et al. "Two New Sulfated Furostanol Saponins From Tribulus Terrestris," *Zeitschrift fur Naturforschung. Journal of Biosciences,* Vol. 57, No. 1-2 (Jan.-Feb. 2002); 33-38.

[69] Ganzera, M., et al. "Determination of Steroidal Saponins in Tribulus Terrestris by Reversed-Phase High-Performance Liquid Chromatography and Evaporative Light Scattering Detection," *Journal of Pharmaceutical Sciences,* Vol. 90, No. 11 (Oct. 2001); 1752-1758.

[70] KO, F.N., et al. "Vasorelaxation of Rat Thoracic Aorta Caused by Osthole Isolated From Angelica Pubescens," *European Journal of Pharmacology,* Vol. 219, No. 1 (Aug. 1992); 29-34.

[71] Chiou, W. F., et al. "Vasorelaxing Effect of Coumarins From Cnidium Monnieri on Rabbit Corpus Cavernosum," *Planta Medica,* Vol. 67, No. 3 (April 2001); 282-284.

[72] Chen, J., et al. "Effect of the Plant-Extract Osthole on the Relaxation of Rabbit Corpus Cavernosum Tissue in Vitro," *Journal of Urology,* Vol. 163, No. 6 (June 2000); 1975-1980.

[73] Jiwajinda, S., et al. "In Vitro Anti-Tumor Promoting and Anti-Parasitic Activities of the Quassinoids from Eurycoma Longifolia, a Medicinal Plant in Southeast Asia," *Journal of Ethnopharmacology,* Vol. 82, No. 1 (Sept. 2002); 55-58.

[74] Kuo, P. C. "Cytotoxic and Antimalarial Constituents From the Roots of Eurycoma Longifolia," *Bioorganic & Medicinal Chemistry,* Vol. 12, No. 3 (Feb. 2004); 537-544.

75   Lin, K.W. "Ethnobotanical Study of Medicinal Plants Used by the Jah Hut Peoples in Malaysia," *Indian Journal of Medical Sciences,* Vol. 59, No. 4 (April 2005); 156-161.

76   Ang, H. H., et al. "Eurycoma Longifolia Jack Enhances Sexual Motivation in Middle-Aged Male Mice," *Journal of Basic and Clinical Physiology and Pharmacology,* Vol. 14, No. 3 (Jan. 2003); 301-308.

77   ———. "Effects of Eurycoma Longifolia Jack (Tongkat Ali) on the Initiation of Sexual Performance of Inexperienced Castrated Male Rats," *Experimental Animals / Japanese Association for Laboratory Animal Science,* Vol. 49, No. 1 (2000); 35-38.

78   ———. "Effect of Eurycoma Longifolia Jack on Orientation Activities in Middle-Aged Male Rats," *Fundamental & Clinical Pharmacology,* Vol. 16 (Dec. 2002); 479.

79   ———. "Eurycoma Longifolia Jack Enhances Libido in Sexually Experienced Male Rats," *Experimental Animals / Japanese Association for Laboratory Animal Science,* Vol. 46, No. 4 (Oct. 1997); 287-290.

80   ———. "Eurycoma Longifolia Increases Sexual Motivation in Sexually Naive Male Rats," *Archives of Pharmacal Research,* Vol. 21, No. 6 (Dec. 1998); 779-781.

81   ———. "Effects of Eurycoma Longifolia Jack on Laevator Ani Muscle in Both Uncastrated and Testosterone-Stimulated Castrated Intact Male Rats," *Archives of Pharmacal Research,* Vol. 24, No. 5 (Oct. 2001); 437-440.

82   Berg A., et al. "Effect of an Oat Bran Enriched Diet on the Atherogenic Lipid Profile in Patients With an Increased Coronary Heart Disease Risk. A Controlled Randomized Lifestyle Intervention Study," *Annals of Nutrition & Metabolism,* Vol. 47 (2003); 306-311.

83   Anderson, J. W., et al. "Oat-Bran Cereal Lowers Serum Total and LDL Cholesterol in Hypercholesterolemic Men," *American Journal of Clinical Nutrition,* Vol. 52 (Dec. 1990); 495-499.

84   Ripson, C. M., et al. "Oat Products and Lipid Lowering. A Meta-Analysis," *The Journal of the American Medical Association,* Vol. 267, No. 24 (June 1992); 3317-3325.

85   Nuengchamnong, N., et al. "HPLC Coupled On-Line to ESI-MS and a DPPH-Based Assay for the Rapid Identification of Anti-Oxidants in Butea Superba," *Phytochemical Analysis,* Vol. 16, No. 6 (Sept. 2005); 422-428.

86   Cherdshewasart, W., et al. "Clinical Trial of Butea Superba, an Alternative Herbal Treatment for Erectile Dysfunction," *Asian Journal of Andrology,* Vol. 5, No.3 (Sept. 2003); 243–246.

87   Moerman, K.L., et al. "Evidence That the Lichen-Derived Scabrosin Esters Target Mitochondrial ATP Synthase in P388D1 Cells," *Toxicology and Applied Pharmacology,* Vol. 190, No. 3 (Aug. 2003); 232-240.

88 Ernst-Russell, M.A., et al. "Structure Revision and Cytotoxic Activity of the Scabrosin Esters, Epidithiopiperazinediones from the Lichen Xanthoparmelia Scabrosa," *Australian Journal of Chemistry,* Vol. 52, No. 4 (1999); 279-283.

89 Kletter, C., et al. "Morphological, Chemical and Functional Analysis of Catuaba Preparations," *Planta Medica,* Vol. 70, No. 10 (Oct. 2004); 993-1000.

90 Lebrett, T., et al. "Efficacy and Safety of a Novel Combination of L-Arginine Glutamate and Yohimbine Hydrochloride: a New Oral Therapy for Erectile Dysfunction," *European Urology,* Vol. 41, No. 6 (June 2002); 608-613.

91 Armanini, D., et al. "Reduction of Serum Testosterone in Men by Licorice," *New England Journal of Medicine,* Vol. 341, No. 15 (Oct. 1999); 1158, (Correspondence).

92 Armanini, D., "Licorice Consumption and Serum Testosterone in Healthy Man," *Experimental and Clinical Endocrinology and Diabetes,* Vol. 111, No.6 (Sept. 2003); 341-343.

93 Josephs, R. A., et al. "Liquorice Consumption and Salivary Testosterone Concentrations," *The Lancet,* Vol. 358 No. 9293 (Nov. 2001); 1613-1614.

94 Fukui, M., et al. "Glycyrrhizin and Serum Testosterone Concentrations in Male Patients With Type 2 Diabetes," *Diabetes Care,* Vol. 26 (2003); 2962, Letter.

95 Verhamme, K., et al. "Nonsteroidal Anti-inflammatory Drugs and Increased Risk of Acute Urinary Retention," *Archives of Internal Medicine,* Vol. 165 No. 13 (July 2005).

96 Barnett, G., et al. "Effects of Marijuana on Testosterone in Male Subjects," *Journal of Theoretical Biology,* Vol. 104, No. 4 (Oct. 1983); 685-692.

97 Block, R. I., et al. "Effects of Chronic Marijuana Use on Testosterone, Luteinizing Hormone, Follicle Stimulating Hormone, Prolactin and Cortisol in Men and Women," *Drug and Alcohol Dependence,* Vol. 28, No. 2 (Aug. 1991); 121-128.

98 Smith, C. G. "Drug Effects on Male Sexual Function," *Clinical Obstetrics and Gynecology,* Vol. 25, No. 3 (Sept. 1982); 525-531.

99 Cone, E. J., et al. "Acute Effects of Smoking Marijuana on Hormones, Subjective Effects and Performance in Male Human Subjects," *Pharmacology, Biochemistry, and Behavior,* Vol. 24, No. 6 (June 1986); 1749-1754.

100 Friedrich, G., et al. "Serum Testosterone Concentrations in Cannabis and Opiate Users," *Beiträge zur Gerichtlichen Medizin,* Vol. 48 (1990); 57-66.

101 McLeod, A. L., et al. "Myocardial Infarction Following the Combined Recreational Use of Viagra and Cannabis," *Clinical Cardiology,* Vol. 25, No. 3 (March 2002); 133-134.

102 Chacko, J., et al. "Association Between Marijuana Use and Transitional Cell Carcinoma," *Urology,* Vol. 67, No. 1(Jan. 2006); 100-104.

Chapter 10

[1] Teloken, C., et al. "Low Serum Testosterone Levels are Associated with Positive Surgical Margins in Radical Retropubic Prostatectomy: Hypogonadism Represents Bad Prognosis in Prostate Cancer," *The Journal of Urology*, Vol. 174, No. 6 (Dec. 2005); 2178-2180.

[2] Raivio, T., et al. "Reduced Circulating Androgen Bioactivity in Patients with Prostate Cancer," *The Prostate*, Vol. 55, No. 3 (April 2003); 194-198.

[3] Steiner, M. S., et al. "Antiestrogens and Selective Estrogen Receptor Modulators Reduce Prostate Cancer Risk," *World Journal of Urology*, Vol. 21, No. 1 (May 2003); 31-36.

[4] Lee, John, *Natural Progesterone, Multiple Roles of a Remarkable Hormone*, 2nd Ed. (Charlbury, UK:, Jon Carpenter Publishing, Market Street, 1999), p. 114.

[5] *Ibid.*, p. 45, 48-49, 65, 93.

[6] Mercola, J, "Progesterone Cream Can Help Prostate Cancer," *Mercola Newsletter*, Issue 67 (Sept. 1998).

[7] Srilatha, B., et al. "Oestrogen-Aandrogen Crosstalk in the Pathophysiology of Erectile Dysfunction," *Asian Journal of Andrology*, Vol. 5 (Dec. 2003); 307-313.

[8] Cowan L. D. et al. "Breast Cancer Incidence in Women With a History of Progesterone Deficiency," *American Journal of Epidemiology*, Vol. 114, No.2 (1981); 209-217.

[9] Morales, A., et al. "Endocrine Aspects of Sexual Dysfunction in Men," *The Journal of Sexual Medicine*, Vol. 1, No. 1 (July 2004).

[10] Reiter, W. J., et al. "Dehydroepiandrosterone in the Treatment of Erectile Dysfunction in Patients with Different Organic Etiologies," *Urological Research*, Vol. 29, No. 4 (Aug. 2001); 278-281.

[11] Williams, M., et al. "Dehydroepiandrosterone Inhibits Human Vascular Smooth Muscle Cell Proliferation Independent of ARs and Ers," *The Journal of Clinical Endocrinology & Metabolism*, Vol. 87, No. 1 (Jan. 2002); 176-181.

[12] Williams, M., et al. "Dehydroepiandrosterone Increases Endothelial Cell Proliferation in Vitro and Improves Endothelial Function in Vivo by Mechanisms Independent of Androgen and Estrogen Receptors," *The Journal of Clinical Endocrinology & Metabolism*, Vol. 89, No. 9 (Sept. 2004); 4708-4715.

[13] Kawano, H., et al. "Dehydroepiandrosterone Supplementation Improves Endothelial Function and Insulin Sensitivity in Men," *The Journal of Clinical Endocrinology & Metabolism*, Vol. 88, No. 7 (July 2003); 3190-3195.

[14] Reiter, W. J. "Dehydroepiandrosterone in the Treatment of Erectile Dysfunction: a Prospective, Double-Blind Randomized, Placebo-Controlled Study," *Urology*, Vol. 53, No. 3 (March 1999); 590-595.

[15] Baulieu, E., et al. "Dehydroepiandrosterone (DHEA), DHEA Sulfate, and Aging: Contribution of the DHEAge Study to a Sociobiomedical Issue," *Proceedings of the National Academy of Sciences,* Vol. 97, No. 8 (April 2000); 4279-4284.

[16] Morales, A., et al. "The Effect of Six Months Treatment With a 100 mg Daily Dose of Dehydroepiandrosterone (DHEA) on Circulating Sex Steroids, Body Composition and Muscle Strength in Age-Advanced Men and Women," *Clinical Endocrinology,* Vol. 49, No. 4 (Oct. 1998); 421-432.

[17] Feldman, H. A., et al. "Massachusetts Male Aging Study," *Journal of Urology,* Vol. 151, No. 1 (Jan. 1994); 54-61.

[18] Baulieu, E., et al. "Dehydroepiandrosterone (DHEA), DHEA Sulfate, and Aging: Contribution of the DHEAge Study to a Sociobiomedical Issue," *Proceedings of the National Academy of Sciences of the United States of America,* Vol. 97, No. 8 (April 2000); 4279-4284.

[19] Rao, K. V. N., et al. "Chemoprevention of Rat Prostate Carcinogenesis by Early and Delayed Administration of Dehydroepiandrosterone," *Cancer Research,* Vol. 59, No. 13 (July 1999); 3084-3089.

[20] Simoncini, T., et al. "Dehydroepiandrosterone Modulates Endothelial Nitric Oxide Synthesis Via Direct Genomic and Nongenomic Mechanisms," *Endocrinology,* Vol. 144, No. 8 (May 2003); 3449-3455.

[21] Williams, M., et al. "Dehydroepiandrosterone Inhibits Human Vascular Smooth Muscle Cell Proliferation Independent of ARs and Ers," *The Journal of Clinical Endocrinology & Metabolism,* Vol. 87, No. 1 (2002); 176-181.

[22] Kawano, H., et al. "Dehydroepiandrosterone Supplementation Improves Endothelial Function and Insulin Sensitivity in Men," *The Journal of Clinical Endocrinology & Metabolism,* Vol. 88, No. 7 (April 2003); 3190-3195.

[23] Villareal, D., et al. Effect of DHEA on Abdominal Fat and Insulin Action in Elderly Women and Men," *Journal of the American Medical Association,* Vol. 292, No. 18 (Nov. 2004); 2243-2248.

[24] Leder, B., et al. "Oral Androstenedione Administration and Serum Testosterone Concentrations in Young Men," *Journal of the American Medical Association,* Vol. 283, No. 6 (Feb. 2000); 779-782.

[25] Kachhi, P., "Priapism after Androstenedione Intake for Athletic Performance Enhancement," *Annals of Emergency Medicine,* Vol. 35, No. 4 (April 2000); 391-393.

[26] Broeder, C,. et al. "The Andro Project: Physiological and Hormonal Influences of Androstenedione Supplementation in Men 35 to 65 Years Old Participating in a High-Intensity Resistance Training Program," *Archives of Internal Medicine,* Vol. 160, No. 20 (Nov. 2000); 3093-3104.

[27] Shores, M. et al. "Low Serum Testosterone and Mortality in Male Veterans," *Archives of Internal Medicine,* Vol. 166, No. 15 (Aug. 2006); 1660-1665.

28   Stattin, P., et al. "High Levels of Circulating Testosterone Are Not Associated with Increased Prostate Cancer Risk: a Pooled Prospective Study," *International Journal of Cancer*, Vol. 108, No. 3 (Oct. 2003); 418-424.

29   Kravchick, S. et al. "Predictive Criteria for Prostate Cancer Detection in Men with Serum PSA Concentration of 2.0 to 4.0 ng/Ml," *Urology*, Vol. 66, No. 3 (Sept. 2005); 542-546.

30   Severi, G., et al. "Circulating Steroid Hormones and the Risk of Prostate Cancer," *Cancer Epidemiology Biomarkers & Prevention*, Vol. 15, No. 1 (Jan. 2006); 86-91.

31   Morales, A. "Androgen Replacement Therapy and Prostate Safety," *European Urology*, Vol. 41, No. 2 (Feb. 2002); 113-120.

32   Parsons, J. K., et al. "Serum Testosterone and the Risk of Prostate Cancer: Potential Implications for Testosterone Therapy," *Cancer Epidemiology Biomarkers & Prevention*, Vol. 14, No. 9 (Sept. 2005); 2257-2260.

33   Barqawi, A., et al. "Testosterone Replacement Therapy and the Risk of Prostate Cancer. Is There a Link?" *International Journal of Impotence Research*, Vol. 18, No. 4 (July 2006); 323-328.

34   Hoffman, M., et al. "Is Low Serum Free Testosterone a Marker for High Grade Prostate Cancer?" *Journal of Urology*, Vol. 163, No. 3 (March 2000); 824-827.

35   Marks, L., et al. "Effects of Testosterone Administration on Prostate Tissues in Men with ADAM Syndrome." Paper presented at the Annual Meeting of the American Urological Association, Atlanta, Georgia, May 2006.

36   Shores, M. M., et al. "Increased Incidence of Diagnosed Depressive Illness in Hypogonadal Older Men," *Archives of General Psychiatry*, Vol. 61, No. 2 (Feb. 2004); 162-167.

37   Fukui, M., et al. "Association Between Serum Testosterone Concentration and Carotid Atherosclerosis in Men With Type 2 Diabetes," *Diabetes Care*, Vol. 26, No. 6 (June 2003); 1869-1873.

38   Travison, T., et al. "The Relationship Between Libido and Testosterone Levels in Aging Men," *The Journal of Clinical Endocrinology & Metabolism*, Vol. 91, No. 7 (July 2006); 2509-2513.

39   Moffat, S. D., et al. "Free Testosterone and Risk for Alzheimer Disease in Older Men," *Neurology*, Vol. 62, No. 2 (Jan. 2004); 188-193.

40   Ding, E. L., et al. "Sex Differences of Endogenous Sex Hormones and Risk of Type 2 Diabetes," *Journal of the American Medical Association*, Vol. 295 No. 11 (March 2006); 1288-1299.

41   Ferrucci, L. et al. "Low Testosterone Levels and the Risk of Anemia in Older Men and Women," *Archives of Internal Medicine*, Vol. 166, No. 13 (July 2006); 1380-1388.

42   Carani, C., et al. "Testosterone and Erectile Function, Nocturnal Penile Tumescence and Rigidity, and Erectile Response to Visual Erotic Stimuli in Hypogonadal and Eugonadal Men," *Psychoneuroendocrinology*, Vol. 17, No. 6 (Nov. 1992); 647-654.

[43] Mills, T., et al. "Androgens and Penile Erection: A Review," *Journal of Anthology,* Vol. 17, No. 6 Nov.-Dec. 1996).

[44] Lee, John, "The John Lee Medical Letter," (March 2002).

[45] Vermeulen, A. "Androgen Replacement Therapy in the Aging Male—A Critical Evaluation," *The Journal of Clinical Endocrinology & Metabolism,* Vol. 86, No. 6 (March 2001); 2380-2390.

[46] Prehn, R. T. "On the Prevention and Therapy of Prostate Cancer by Androgen Administration," *Cancer Research,* Vol. 59 (Sept. 1999); 4161-4164.

Chapter 11

[1] Donaldson, M. "Nutrition and Cancer — A Review of the Evidence for an Anti-Cancer Diet," *Nutrition Journal,* Vol. 3:19 (Oct. 2004).

[2] Heaney, R. "Long-Latency Deficiency Disease: Insights From Calcium and Vitamin D," *American Journal of Clinical Nutrition,* Vol. 78, No. 5 (Nov. 2003); 912-919.

[3] Fleshner, N., et al. "Diet, Androgens, Oxidative Stress and Prostate Cancer Susceptibility," *Cancer Metastasis Review,* Vol. 17, No. 4 (Dec. 1998); 325-330.

[4] Ornish, D., et al. "Intensive Lifestyle Changes May Affect The Progression of Prostate Cancer," *Journal of Urology,* Vol. 174, No. 3 (Sept. 2005); 1065-1070.

[5] Esposito, K., et al. "Effect of Lifestyle Changes on Erectile Dysfunction in Obese Men," *Journal of the American Medical Association,* Vol. 291, No. 24 (June 2004).

[6] Ganmaa, D., et al. "A Two-Generation Reproduction Study to Assess the Effects of Cows' Milk on Reproductive Development in Male and Female Rats," *Fertility and Sterility,* Vol. 82, No. 3 (Oct. 2004); 1106-1114.

[7] Ganmaa, D., et al. "Commercial Cows' Milk Has Uterotrophic Activity on the Uteri of Young Ovariectomized Rats and Immature Rats," *International Journal of Cancer,* Vol. 118, No. 9 (May 2006); 2363-2365.

[8] Cross, A., et al. "A Prospective Study of Meat and Meat Mutagens and Prostate Cancer Risk," *Cancer Research,* Vol. 65, No. 24 (Dec. 2005); 11779-11784.

[9] DeMarzo, A. "Charred Meats Tied to Prostate Cancer." American Association of Cancer Research, Annual Meeting, Washington (April 2006).

[10] Pelucci, C., et al. "Fibre Intake and Prostate Cancer Risk," *International Journal of Cancer,* Vol. 109, No. 2 (March 2004); 278-280.

[11] Millett, C., et al. "Smoking and Erectile Dysfunction: Findings From a Representative Sample of Australian Men," *Tobacco Control,* Vol. 15 (April 2006); 136-139.

[12] Gades, N., et al. "Association Between Smoking and Erectile Dysfunction: A Population-Based Study," *American Journal of Epidemiology,* Vol. 161, No. 4 (Feb. 2005); 346-351.

[13] Verhamme, K., et al. "Nonsteroidal Anti-inflammatory Drugs and Increased Risk of Acute Urinary Retention," *Archives of Internal Medicine*, Vol. 165, No. 13 (July 2005).

[14] Bairati, I., et al. "Lifetime Occupational Physical Activity and Incidental Prostate Cancer," *Cancer Causes Control*, Vol. 11, No. 8 (Sept. 2000); 759-764.

[15] Friedenreich, C., et al. "Case-Control Study of Lifetime Total Physical Activity and Prostate Cancer Risk," *American Journal of Epidemiology*, Vol. 159, No. 8 (April 2004); 740-749.

[16] Giovannucci, E., et al. "A Prospective Study of Physical Activity and Incident and Fatal Prostate Cancer," *Archives of Internal Medicine*, Vol. 165, No. 9 (May 2005); 1005-1010.

[17] Oliveria, S., et al. "Is Exercise Beneficial in the Prevention of Prostate Cancer?" *Sports Medicine*, Vol. 23, No. 5 (May 1997); 271-278.

[18] Oliveria, S., et al. "The Association Between Cardiorespiratory Fitness and Prostate Cancer," *Medicine & Science in Sports & Exercise*, Vol. 28, No. 1 (Jan. 1996); 97-104.

[19] Tymchuk, C., et al. "Effects of Diet and Exercise on Insulin, Sex Hormone-Binding Globulin, and Prostate-Specific Antigen," *Nutrition and Cancer*, Vol. 31, No. 2 (1998); 127-131.

[20] Bacon, C., et al. "Sexual Function in Men Older Than 50 Years of Age: Results from the Health Professionals Follow-up Study," *Annals of Internal Medicine*, Vol. 139, No. 3 (Aug. 2003); 161-168.

[21] Derby, C., et al. "Modifiable Risk Factors and Erectile Dysfunction: Can Lifestyle Changes Modify Risk?" *Urology*, Vol. 56, No. 2 (Aug. 2000); 302-306.

[22] Oremek, G. et al. "Physical Activity Releases Prostate-Specific Antigen (PSA) From the Prostate Gland Into Blood and Increases Serum PSA Concentrations," *Clinical Chemistry*, Vol. 42, No. 5 (May 1996); 691-695.

[23] Kubo, T., et al. "Prospective Cohort Study of the Risk of Prostate Cancer Among Rotating-Shift Workers: Findings from the Japan Collaborative Cohort Study," *American Journal of Epidemiology*, Vol. 164, No. 6 (Sept. 2006); 549-555.

[24] Stevens, V., et al. "Folate Nutrition and Prostate Cancer Incidence in a Large Cohort of US Men," *American Journal of Epidemiology*, Vol.163, No. 11 (June 2006); 989-996.

[25] Eussen, S., et al. "Oral Cyanocobalamin Supplementation in Older People With Vitamin B12 Deficiency," *Archives of Internal Medicine*, Vol. 165 No. 10 (May 2005); 1167-1172.

[26] Barry, M. J., et al. "The American Urological Association Symptom Index For Benign Prostatic Hyperplasia," *Journal of Urology*, Vol. 148, No. 5 (Nov. 1992); 1549-1557.

27 Jankowska, E. A., et al. "Anabolic Deficiency in Men with Chronic Heart Failure," *Circulation,* Vol. 114 (Oct. 2006); 1829-1837.

28 Orwoll, E., et al. "Endogenous Testosterone Levels, Physical Performance, and Fall Risk in Older Men," *Archives of Internal Medicine,* Vol. 166 No. 19 (Oct. 2006); 2124-2131.

29 Huggins, C., et al. "The Effects of Castration on Advanced Carcinoma of the Prostate Gland," *Archives of Surgery,* Vol. 43 (1941); 209.

30 Banks, J., et al. "Disease and Disadvantage in the United States and in England," *Journal of the American Medical Association.*

Glossary

5-Alpha-Reductase — An enzyme that converts the male sex hormone, testosterone, into its more active form, dihydrotestosterone. High levels of this enzyme can cause excessive prostate tissue growth.

Adaptogen — An herbal agent that helps the body normalize its processes without adverse effects.

ADT — Androgen Deprivation Therapy — A drug treatment used for metastatic prostate cancer.

Anorgasmia — Inability to have a normal orgasm even with adequate stimulation. A common cause of anorgasmia in older men is hormone imbalances, particularly low free testosterone levels. Other causes are various medications for BPH, antidepressant medications, and deterioration of nerve sensitivity due to underlying medical conditions like diabetes.

Antioxidants — Substances that reduce or eliminate the rate of oxidation caused by free radicals in the body. Plant products contain an abundant variety of different antioxidants.

Apoptosis — The process that enables unneeded or defective individual cells to commit suicide. Also called programmed cell death.

Aphrodisiac — A food, herb, or other substance that has a reputed ability to intensify sexual desire.

Arteriosclerosis — Thickening, toughening, stiffening, and loss of elasticity of the arteries due to aging or disease. Typically known as "hardening of the arteries." Also called atherosclerosis.

Aromatase — An enzyme that converts testosterone to estrogen. Herbs that inhibit aromatase can help reduce estrogen levels and increase testosterone levels.

Atherosclerosis — The progressive narrowing of arteries due to deposits of cholesterol and other substances on the inner walls. Sometimes also called arteriosclerosis.

Bio-identical — Substances that are identical to those produced naturally by the body.

BPH — Benign prostate hyperplasia or benign prostate hypertrophy — is an enlargement of the prostate gland typically affecting aging men. The enlarged prostate constricts the urethra causing urinary problems ranging from minor annoyances to serious medical problems.

Capillaries — Minute, hair-like blood vessels found throughout the body and particularly abundant in the prostate.

Castration — The process of rendering the testicles, and the androgen hormones they produce, inactive. It can be done pharmaceutically with certain drugs, or it can involve surgical removal of the testicles (orchiectomy). It is usually used as a treatment for metastatic prostate cancer.

Carcinogens — Chemical items or irritants known to cause cancer.

Cialis® — Tadalafil — A prescription erectile dysfunction drug.

Circadian Rhythm — A repetitive 24-hour cycle that occurs in most mammals and plants. Also called circadian clock or circadian pattern.

Corpora cavernosa/Corpora spongiosa — The highly expandable sponge-like tissue that runs the entire length of the penis. An erection occurs when this tissue fills with blood.

CVD — Cardiovascular Disease — A general term for a group of conditions that involve the blood vessels and the heart and result in impaired blood circulation throughout the body.

Endocrine system — A body system consisting of several glands that secrete hormones into the bloodstream.

Endothelial tissue — The thin flat layer of cells that lines all blood vessels in the body. Endothelial dysfunction is directly associated with atherosclerosis, cardiovascular disease, erectile dysfunction, and other circulatory problems.

Enzyme — a protein that acts as an organic catalyst and is able to initiate or accelerate a specific biochemical reaction in the body.

Erectile Dysfunction — Inability to maintain an erection sufficient for normal intercourse.

Estrogen — For the purposes of this book, the term "estrogen" is used to refer to the group of predominantly female hormones consisting of estradiol, estrone, and estriol.

Etiology — Generally refers to the cause or causes of a disease or dysfunction.

Free Radicals — Chemically, free radicals are molecules with unpaired electrons that are usually highly reactive and very likely to participate in chemical reactions. They are produced as a result of normal metabolism and can cause damage to cells if they are not neutralized and removed quickly. See antioxidants.

Gynecomastia — Excessive enlargement of male breasts. Can be due to an overabundance of estrogens and a low level of free testosterone. A side effect of some drugs used for BPH and ADT.

Herbalist — A person knowledgeable in the properties of herbs for general and medicinal purposes.

Homeostasis — The ability of the human body to adjust its internal processes for the purpose of maintaining itself in balance.

Hypertension — High blood pressure. Defined as a chronic elevation in blood pressure over 140/90.

IIEF — International Index of Erectile Function — A questionnaire that yields a rough indication of the degree of erectile dysfunction.

IPSS — International Prostate Symptom Score — A questionnaire that yields a rough indication of the degree of prostate dysfunction. Useful to track changes over time.

Impotence — A synonym for Erectile Dysfunction. Generally an older term.

Ischemia — A shortage of oxygen due to insufficient blood flow. Ischemic heart disease is a condition caused by a decrease in blood supply to the heart, usually by constriction or obstruction of the arteries leading to the heart.

JAMA — Journal of the American Medical Association.

Levitra® — Vardenafil. — A prescription erectile dysfunction drug.

Libido — Level of desire for sexual intimacy. Highly linked to levels of free testosterone in both men and women.

Meta-analysis — In medicine, a statistical analysis of many separate but related medical studies.

Metabolism — The process by which the body produces energy from the chemical breakdown of ingested nutrients.

Micronutrients — Vitamins, minerals, and other food substances essential for good health in extremely small amounts.

Nocturnal — During the night.

Nutrients — Elements that provide the body with the fuel it needs to generate energy and function.

ODA or ODR — Optimal Daily Allowance or Optimal Daily Requirement.

Osteoporosis — A disease of the bone that results in reduced bone mass and increased risk of fractures. In older men, it can be exacerbated by testosterone deficiencies.

Phytochemicals — A general term for chemicals produced by all plants.

Phytoestrogens — Chemicals found in plants that mimic the effects of estrogen in the human body.

Phytonutrients — Nutrients found in plants and plant products.

Phytosterols — Plant fats that are chemically similar to cholesterol. Also known as sterols and sterolins.

Priapism — An unwanted, and sometimes painful erection of excessive duration. Priapism in excess of several hours may need surgical intervention.

Prostatectomy — Surgical removal of all or part of the prostate gland.

PSA (prostate-specific antigen) — A protein manufactured exclusively by the prostate gland that is often used as a marker for prostate disease. High levels usually are associated with prostate dysfunction, often prostate cancer.

Pseudoestrogens — Also known as *xenoestrogens* — Terms coined by various researchers to describe chemicals in our environment and food chain that produce estrogen-like effects on the body.

RDA — Recommended Dietary Allowance (or RDI — Recommended Daily Intake) — A value set by the U.S. Department of Agriculture as the daily intake level of a nutrient considered needed by most individuals. This is the reference for the values printed on food labels in the U.S. and Canada. See ODA.

SHBG — Sex hormone binding globulin — A protein that binds to testosterone reducing levels of free testosterone.

Synergy — The result of two or more substances acting together that produces an effect greater than that expected from either substance acting alone.

Testicular atrophy — Shrinking of the testicles. Can be due to excess estrogen or low testosterone.

Triglycerides — Fatty acids in the blood. High triglyceride levels often coincide with high cholesterol levels.

Urethra — The tube that channels urine and semen out of the body through the penis.

USP — An acronym for United States Pharmaceutical. Indicates a pharmaceutical grade product.

Vasectomy — A surgical procedure typically used as a method of male sterilization that removes part of the vas deferens and eliminates the path for semen to leave the body through the penis.

Vas deferens —The tubes that carry sperm cells from the testicles to the ejaculatory ducts. Cutting the vas deferens results in male sterilization. See Vasectomy.

Vascular — Relating to the vessels that carry fluids like blood and lymph through the body.

Vascular insufficiency — A more precise term used for impaired blood circulation.

Viagra® — Sildenafil citrate — A prescription erectile dysfunction drug.

Xenoestrogens — See Pseudoestrogens.

Bibliography

Balch, James, M.D., *Prescription for Nutritional Healing, 3rd Ed.* Avery, New York, NY, 2000.

Ballentine, Robert, M.D., *Diet and Nutrition.* Honesdale, PA, Himalayan Institute Press, 1978.

Bartram, Thomas, *Bartram's Encyclopedia of Natural Medicine.* New York: Marlowe & Company, 1995.

Bonnard, Marc, M.D., *The Viagra Alternative.* Rochester, VT.: Healing Arts Press, 1999.

Castleman, Michael. *The New Healing Herbs.* New York: Bantam, 2002.

Clapp, Larry, Ph.D., *Prostate Health in 90 Days.* Carlsbad, CA.: Hay House, 1997.

Duke, James, Ph.D., *Herbs of the Bible.* Loveland, CO.: Interweave press, 1999.

Duke, James, Ph.D., *The Green Pharmacy.* New York: St. Martin's Press, 1997.

Faigin, Rob, J.D., *Natural Hormone Enhancement.* Cedar Mountain, NC.: Extique Publishing, 2000.

Falcone, Ron, *Natural Medicine for Prostate Problems.* New York: Dell Publishing, 1998.

Goldberg, Burton. *Alternative Medicine - The Definitive Guide.* Tiburon, CA.: Future Medicine Publishing, 1997.

Hobday, Richard. *The Healing Sun: Sunlight and Health in the 21st Century.* Findhorn, Scotland, 2000.

Hoffer, Abram, M.D., Ph.D., *Putting it all Together.* New Canaan, CT.: Keats Publishing, 1996.

Hoffer, Abram, M.D., Ph.D., *Vitamin C and Cancer: Discovery, Recovery, Controversy.* Kingston, Ontario, Canada: Quarry Health Books Press, SCB Distributors, 2001.

Jensen, Bernard, Ph.D., *The Chemistry of Man.* Escondido, CA.: Bernard Jensen International, 1983.

Kaltenbach, Don, *Prostate Cancer – A Survivor's Guide.* Sarasota, FL.: Seneca House Press, 2003.

Lee, John, M.D., *Natural Progesterone: The multiple roles of a remarkable hormone.* Second Ed. Charlbury, U.K.: Jon Carpenter Publishing, 2002.

———. *What Your Doctor May Not Tell You About Breast Cancer.* New York: Warner Books, 2002.

———. *What Your Doctor May Not Tell You About Premenopause.* New York: Warner Books, 1996.

———. *What Your Doctor May Not Tell You About Menopause.* New York: Warner Books, 1999.

Lepore, Donald, N.D., N.M.D., *The Ultimate Healing System.* Orem, UT.: Woodland Publishing, 1985.

Lininger, Schuyler, D.C., *The Natural Pharmacy, 2nd Ed.,* New York: Prima Publishing,1999.

Loomis, Howard F., D.C., *Enzymes, The Key to Health.* Madison, WI: 21st Century Nutrition Publishing,1999.

Love, Susan, M.D., *Dr. Susan Love's Breast Book.* Menlo Park, CA: Addison-Wesley Publishing, 1991.

Maleskey, Gale. *Nature's Medicines.* Emmaus, PA: Prevention Health Books, Rodale Press,1999.

Mason, Roger. *The Natural Prostate Cure.* East Canaan, CT: Safe Goods, 2000.

Mindell, Earl, R.Ph., Ph.D. *New Herb Bible.* New York: Simon & Schuster, 2000.

Morganstern, Steven, M.D. *The Prostate Sourcebook.* Los Angeles, CA: Lowell House, 1994.

Murray, Michael, N.D. *Encyclopedia of Natural Medicine.* Rockland, CA: Prima Publishing, 1998.

Murray, Michael, N.D. *How to Prevent and Treat Cancer with Natural Medicine.* New York: Riverhead Books, 2002.

Murray, Michael, N.D. *Male Sexual Vitality.* Rockland, CA: Prima Publishing, 1994.

Netzer, Corinne. *The Complete Book of Food Counts.* New York: Dell Publishing, 2000.

Netzer, Corinne. *The Complete Book of Vitamin and Mineral Counts.* New York: Dell Publishing, 1997.

Null, Gary, Ph.D. *The Complete Encyclopedia of Natural Healing.* New York: Kensington Books, 1998.

Pederson, Mark, N.D. *Nutritional Herbology.* Warsaw, IN.: W.W. Whitman Co, 1998.

Plotkin, Mark, Ph.D. *Medicine Quest.* New York: Penguin Books, 2000.

Redmon, George, Ph.D., N.D. *Managing and Preventing Prostate Disorders.* Prescott, AZ: Hohm Press, 2000.

Ricketts, David. *Eat to Beat Prostate Cancer Cookbook.* New York: Harry N. Abrams, Inc., STC Healthy Living, 2006.

Ritchason, Jack, N.D. *The Little Herb Encyclopedia.* Pleasant Grove, UT: Woodland Books, 1995.

Roberts, H. J., M.D. *Is Vasectomy Worth the Risk? A Physician's Case Against Vasectomania.* West Palm Beach, FL.: Sunshine Sentinel Press, 1993.

Rouse, Stephen, M.D. *The Prostate Book.* New York: W. W. Norton & Company, 1992.

Rubin, Jordan, N.M.D., Ph.D. *The Maker's Diet.* Lake Mary, FL.: Strang Communications, 2004.

Shippen, Eugene, M.D. *The Testosterone Syndrome.* New York: M. Evans & Co, 1998.

Stoff, Jesse, M.D. *The Prostate Miracle.* New York: Kensington, 1995.

Tierra, Michael, N.D. *Planetary Herbology.* Twin Lakes, WI: Lotus Press, 1992.

Walsh, Patrick, M.D. *Guide to Surviving Prostate Cancer.* New York: Warner Books, 2001.

Weil, Andrew, M.D. *Eating Well for Optimal Health.* New York: A. A. Knopf Publishing, 2000.

————. *Natural Health, Natural Medicine.* Boston: Houghton Miffin Co., 1998.

————. *Spontaneous Healing.* New York: Ballantine, 2000.

White, Linda, M.D. *The Herbal Drugstore.* New York: Signet Health Books, 2002.

Young, Robert, Ph.D. *The pH Miracle.* New York: Warner Books, 2002.

Index